The Art & Science of Nurse Coaching

The Provider's Guide to Coaching Scope and Competencies

Darlene R. Hess PhD, RN, AHN-BC, PMHNP-BC, ACC, HWNC-BC
Director, Brown Mountain Visions, Los Ranchos, New Mexico
Faculty, University of Phoenix, Albuquerque, New Mexico
Faculty, Northern New Mexico College, Espanola, New Mexico
Committee Member, National Consortium for Credentialing of Health and Wellness Coaches

Barbara M. Dossey, PhD, RN, AHN-BC, FAAN, HWNC-BC
Co-Director, International Nurse Coach Association
Core Faculty, Integrative Nurse Coach Certificate Program, Huntington, New York
International Co-Director, Nightingale Initiative for Global Health, Washington, DC and Neepewa, Manitoba, Canada
Director, Holistic Nursing Consultants, Santa Fe, New Mexico
Committee Member, National Consortium for Credentialing of Health and Wellness Coaches

Mary Elaine Southard, MSN, RN, AHN-BC, CHOM, HWNC-BC
Director, Integrative Health Consulting and Coaching, LLC, Scranton, Pennsylvania
Board Member, American Holistic Nurses Credentialing Corporation (AHNCC), Cedar Park, Texas
Committee Member, National Consortium for Credentialing of Health and Wellness Coaches

Susan Luck, MA, RN, HNB-BC, CCN, HWNC-BC
Co-Director, International Nurse Coach Association
Core Faculty, Integrative Nurse Coach Certificate Program, Huntington, New York
Director, EarthRose Institute for Environmental Health, Miami, Florida
Faculty, University of Miami, Clinical Nutrition Program, Department of Family Medicine, Miami, Florida
Committee Member, National Consortium for Credentialing of Health and Wellness Coaches

Bonney Gulino Schaub, MS, RN, PMHCNS-BC, NC-BC
Co-Director, International Nurse Coach Association
Core Faculty, Integrative Nurse Coach Certificate Program
Co-Director and Core Faculty, Huntington Meditation and Imagery Center, Huntington, New York
Committee Member, National Consortium for Credentialing of Health and Wellness Coaches

Linda Bark, PhD, RN, MCC, NC-BC
President, Bark Coaching Institute, Alameda, California
Faculty, JFK Holistic Health Masters Program, Pleasant Hill, California
Faculty/Mentor, National Institute of Whole Health, Boston, Massachusetts
Leadership Team, National Consortium for Credentialing of Health and Wellness Coaches

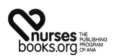
nurses books.org THE PUBLISHING PROGRAM OF ANA

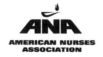
ANA
AMERICAN NURSES ASSOCIATION

Silver Spring, Maryland
2013

Library of Congress Cataloging-in-Publication data

The art and science of nurse coaching : the provider's guide to coaching scope and competencies / Darlene Hess ... [et al.].

   p. ; cm.

 Includes bibliographical references and index.

 ISBN 978-1-55810-494-5 (softcover : alk. paper) -- ISBN 978-1-55810-495-2 (ebook : pdf format) -- ISBN 978-1-55810-496-9 (ebook : epub format) -- ISBN 978-1-55810-497-6 (ebook : mobipocket format)

 I. Hess, Darlene. II. American Nurses Association.

 [DNLM: 1. Mentors--United States. 2. Nurses--United States. 3. Inservice Training--United States. 4. Leadership--United States. 5. Nurse's Role--United States. WY 18]

   610.73--dc23

                          2012048696

The American Nurses Association (ANA) is a national professional association. This ANA publication—*The Art and Science of Nurse Coaching: The Provider's Guide to Coaching Scope and Competencies*—reflects the thinking of registered nurses on various issues and should be reviewed in conjunction with state board of nursing policies and practices. State law, rules, and regulations govern the practice of nursing, while *The Art and Science of Nurse Coaching: The Provider's Guide to Coaching Scope and Competencies* guides registered nurses in the application of their professional skills and responsibilities.

American Nurses Association
8515 Georgia Avenue, Suite 400
Silver Spring, MD 20910-3492
1-800-274-4ANA
http://www.NursingWorld.org

Published by Nursesbooks.org
The Publishing Program of ANA
http://www.Nursesbooks.org/

ISBN: 978-1-55810-494-5   SAN: 851-3481   01/2017R
First printing: January 2013   Second printing: April 2014   Third printing: January 2017

Contents

Contributors

Professional Nurse Coaching Workgroup (PNCW) (2009–2012)

Darlene Hess, PhD, AHN-BC, PMHNP-BC, ACC, HWNC-BC, Co-Chair

Barbara M. Dossey, PhD, RN, AHN-BC, FAAN, HWNC-BC, Co-Chair

Mary Elaine Southard, MSN, RN, AHN-BC, CHOM, HWNC-BC

Susan Luck, MA, RN, HNB-BC, CCN, HWNC-BC

Bonney Gulino Schaub, MS, RN, PMHCNS-BC, NC-BC

Linda Bark, PhD, RN, MCC, NC-BC

Professional Nurse Coaching Review Committee (2011–2012)

Phyllis Kritek, PhD, RN, FAAN, Co-Chair

Barbara L. Nichols, DHL, MS, RN, FAAN, Co-Chair

Denys Cope, BSN, RN

Liz Cunningham, MA, RN

Michelle Dart, MSN, RN, CNE

Gail Donner, PhD, RN

Lori Knutson, BSN, RN, HN-BC

Mary Jo Kreitzer, PhD, RN, FAAN

Kristen Lombard, PhD, RN, PMHCNS-BC

Eileen O'Grady, PhD, RN

Diane Pisanos, MS, RN, NNP-E, AHN-BC

Kimberly McNally, MN, RN

Darlene Trandel, PhD, FNP, RN, PCC

Pat Hinton-Walker, PhD, RN, FAAN, CMC, PCC

Mary Wheeler, MEd, RN, PCC

Linda Yoder, PhD, RN, AOCN, FAAN

Professional Nurse Coaching Advisory Committee (2011–2012)

Daniel J. Pesut, PhD, RN, PMHCNS-BC, FAAN, Co-Chair

Jean Watson, PhD, RN, FAAN, Co-Chair

Patricia Benner, PhD, RN, FAAN

Nancy Dickerson-Hazard, MSN, RN, CPNP, FAAN

Debra Geradi, MPD, RN, JD

JoEllen Koerner, PhD, RN, FAAN

Mary Jo Kreitzer, PhD, RN, FAAN

Mary Wheeler, MEd, RN, PCC

Beverly Malone, PhD, RN, FAAN

Cheryl A. Peterson, MSN, RN

Franklin A. Shaffer, EdD, RN, FAAN

Endorsing Organizations

The following list is of the endorsing organizations for this document as of December 2012. Other organizations will be added in future editions.

American Academy of Nursing
American Academy of Ambulatory Care Nursing
American Association of Critical Care Nurses
American Holistic Nurses Association
American Holistic Nurses Credentialing Corporation
American Nephrology Nurses Association
American Nurses Association
American Psychiatric Nurses Association
Bark Coaching International
CGFNS International
Emergency Nurses Association
International Association of Human Caring
International Nurse Coach Association
National Gerontological Nursing Association
National League for Nursing
Nurse Organization of Veterans Affairs
Preventive Cardiovascular Nurses Association
Sigma Theta Tau International
Society for the Advancement of Modeling and Role-Modeling
Society of Gastroenterology Nurses and Associates
Watson Caring Science Institute

Preamble

The Art and Science of Nurse Coaching: The Provider's Guide to Coaching Scope and Competencies defines and explains the role of the Nurse Coach within the context of *Nursing: Scope and Standards of Practice*, 2nd Edition (American Nursing Association [ANA], 2010a) and emerging trends in interprofessional health professions education (Interprofessional Education Collaborative Expert Panel, 2011). The International Coach Federation (ICF) Professional Coaching Core Competencies (ICF, 2008a) inform key elements of this document.

The professional Nurse Coach role and coaching are a fundamental part of nursing practice. The professional Nurse Coach role competencies prepare nurses to integrate this role within all specialty areas and settings. Nurse coaching is not a specialty area of nursing practice. Nurse Coaching competencies are based in nursing theories, social and behavioral science theories, and evidence-based promotion of health and well-being. The Nurse Coach uses inquiry and skillfully requests permission to share information instead of coming from an expert role used in patient education and teaching.

Executive Summary

Introduction

There are 3.1 million nurses in the United States (ANA, 2010; American Association of Colleges of Nursing [AACN], 2011) and 17.6 million nurses and midwives in the world (WHO, 2009). The 2010 report from the Institute of Medicine (IOM), *The Future of Nursing* and other health initiatives suggest the need for increased education and leadership from nurses to address the healthcare needs of our nation and world. Nurse Coaches are strategically positioned to skillfully partner with clients to assess, strategize, plan, and evaluate progress towards negotiated coaching goals. Coaching is a natural extension of nursing practice. Professional Nurse Coaches are equipped to implement health-promoting and evidence-based strategies with clients and support behavioral and lifestyle changes to enhance growth, overall health and well-being. With possibilities not yet imagined, employment opportunities for nurses who incorporate coaching into professional practice are developing across the entire spectrum of health, wellness, and healing.

As the healthcare system shifts from a disease-focused and reactive health-care system to one proactively focused on culturally sensitive wellness, health promotion, and disease prevention, the Nurse Coach role is an essential ingredient of success to assist people towards sustained health. Chronic disease, stress-related illnesses, and entrenched unhealthy lifestyles make health, healing, and well-being challenging to attain and sustain. Nurses need to develop skillful means of partnering and collaborating with clients in new ways, which acknowledge clients as experts in their own care.

Purpose

The purpose of *The Art and Science of Nurse Coaching* is to define and clarify the foundation of the Nurse Coach role and demonstrate nursing's leadership and proactive stance in healthcare transformation.

The Art and Science of Nurse Coaching explains nursing perspectives concerning the role of the Nurse Coach in five key ways: (1) It specifies the philosophy, beliefs, and values of the Nurse Coach and the Nurse Coach's scope of practice; (2) It articulates the relationship between *The Art and Science of Nurse Coaching: The Provider's Guide to Coaching Scope and Competencies* and ANA's *Nursing: Scope and Standards of Practice*, 2nd Edition; (3) It provides the basis for continued interdisciplinary conversations related to professional health and wellness coaches and lay health and wellness coaches; (4) It lays the foundation for an international certification process for professional Nurse Coaching practice; and (5) It identifies the need to develop a core curriculum for professional Nurse Coaching practice that can be used in practice, education, research and the development and evaluation of healthcare policy.

Integrated throughout this document is attention to professional nursing philosophy, values, ethics, and beliefs, an artful use of the nursing process, and contemporary interprofessional collaborative conversations (see the note at the end of this section) related to coaching. The audience for this publication expands beyond nursing proper to include interdisciplinary systems, communities and populations.

Process

The Art and Science of Nurse Coaching delineates the efforts of the Professional Nurse Coach Workgroup (PNCW) (see Contributors section, starting on page vii) and is the product of significant exploratory conversations and electronic mail communication among professional Nurse Coaches and nurse leaders that resulted in a six-step process over a three-year period.

During initial meetings fundamental concepts of Nurse Coaching and the Nurse Coach role as a component of nursing practice were analyzed and discussed. These discussions also included considerations related to the growing emergence of nonprofessional health and wellness coaches as well as the development of health and wellness coaches in other professions. In September 2010, the PNCW circulated *White Paper on Holistic Nurse Coaching* (Hess, Bark, & Southard, 2010) at the National Summit on Standards and Credentialing of Professional Coaches in Healthcare and Wellness (NCCHWC) convened by the National Consortium for the Credentialing of Health and Wellness Coaches in Boston, Massachusetts, to explore the future of health and wellness coaches (NCCHWC, 2010; 2011). *The Art and Science of Nurse Coaching: The Provider's Guide to Coaching Scope and Competencies* has been developed by Nurse Coach experts and vetted via a thorough peer-review process to fully describe the professional Nurse Coach role.

The PNCW entered into a conversation regarding the importance of the role of the Nurse Coach and the need for a national certification process for professional Nurse Coaches with the American Holistic Nurse Credentialing Corporation (AHNCC)(Appendix B). After lengthy discussion, the PNCW entered an agreement with AHNCC whereby AHNCC would sponsor the work of the PNCW in exchange for the rights to establish a national certification process for the Nurse Coach. The PNCW remains engaged in conversations related to alliances with other interprofessional organizations for the purpose of establishing clear guidelines and competencies for professional health and wellness coaches.

An in-depth six-step course of action included the completion of an extensive literature review, compilation of the findings, and development of a draft document. The PNCW engaged with an expert Review Committee and an Advisory Committee comprised of Nurse Coaches and leaders (see Contributors section, starting on page vii). After extensive reviews and several revisions by the PNCW members, the draft document was submitted to the committees for comments, deletions, modifications, and recommendations. Additional reviews were completed and led to the development of a revised document that was sent to the American Nurses Association (ANA) December 1, 2011 to begin the steps towards becoming an endorsed ANA document with additional endorsements from professional nursing organizations.

Definitions and Scope of Practice

[Note: The word client *is interchangeable with the word patient throughout this document.]*

The Nurse Coach is a registered nurse who integrates coaching competencies into any setting or specialty area of practice to facilitate a process of change or development that assists individuals or groups to realize their potential. Nurse Coaching is a skilled, purposeful, results-oriented, and structured relationship-centered interaction with clients provided by registered nurses for the purpose of promoting achievement of client goals. The Nurse Coach role has roots in Florence Nightingale's legacy, nursing history and theories and the social sciences.

Nurse Coaching involves the ability to develop a coaching partnership, to create a safe space, and to be sensitive to client issues of trust and vulnerability (Schaub & Schaub, 2009) as a basis for further exploration, self-discovery and action planning related to desired outcomes. Coaching builds on client strengths rather than attempting to "fix" weaknesses. The Nurse Coach must be able to explore client readiness for coaching, structure a coaching session, facilitate achievement of the client's desired goals, and co-create a means of determining and evaluating desired outcomes and goals (Hess, Bark, & Southard, 2010). Nurse Coaching is grounded in the principles and core values of professional nursing.

Nurse Coaches are found in all areas of nursing practice and work with individuals and with groups. Nurse Coaches are staff nurses, ambulatory care nurses, case managers, advanced practice nurses, nursing faculty, nurse researchers, educators, administrators, or nurse entrepreneurs. Nurse Coaches may practice in a specialty area such as diabetes education, cardiac rehabilitation, or end-of-life care.

Nurse Coaches may focus on health and wellness coaching, executive coaching, faculty development coaching, managerial coaching, business coaching, or life coaching. The extent to which registered nurses engage in the Nurse Coach role is dependent on coach-specific education, training, experience, position, and the population they serve.

✕ Professional Nurse Coach Competencies and the Nurse Coaching Process

The Art and Science of Nurse Coaching identifies the Nurse Coach competencies that are linked to each of the ANA six standards of practice (assessment, diagnosis, outcomes identification, planning, implementation, evaluation) and ten standards of professional performance (ethics, education, evidence-based practice and research, quality of practice, communication, leadership, collaboration, professional practice evaluation, resources utilization, environmental health) (ANA, 2010a). A description of the professional Nurse Coach role pertaining to each standard is provided followed by the Specific Nurse Coach Competencies related to that standard.

The professional Nurse Coaching competencies are authoritative statements of the duties that all Nurse Coaches are expected to perform competently, regardless of setting or specialization. The list of competencies is not exhaustive. The contents of this document will be expanded as new and broader patterns of the Nurse Coach role are developed and accepted by the nursing profession. The Nurse Coaching competencies are applicable to all areas of Nurse Coaching practice.

The Nurse Coaching Process is a reorientation of the nursing process.

The Nurse Coaching Process includes six steps as follows: (1) Establishing Relationship and Identifying Readiness for Change (Assessment); (2) Identifying Opportunities, Issues, and Concerns (Diagnosis); (3) Establishing Client-Centered Goals (Outcomes); (4) Creating the Structure of the Coaching Interaction (Plan); (5) Empowering and Motivating Clients to Reach Goals (Intervention); and (6) and Assisting Clients to Determine the Extent to which Goals were Achieved (Evaluation).

Summary of Content

The Art and Science of Nurse Coaching is a comprehensive document that further includes a discussion of:

- Foundational professional nursing documents that guide professional Nurse Coaching practice

- Definition of professional Nurse Coach and professional Nurse Coaching practice

- Professional Nurse Coaching scope of practice

- Nurse Coaching process

- Tenets characteristics of professional Nurse Coaching practice

- Healthy environments (internal and external) for professional Nurse Coaching practice

- ANA standards as organizing framework for professional Nurse Coaching practice

- Professional competence in professional Nurse Coaching practice

- Professional Nurse Coaching practice today

- Professional Nurse Coaching research and evidence-based practice

- Progression of curriculum development, certificate programs, and national certification for professional Nurse Coaching

- IOM influences on professional Nurse Coaching practice and leadership

- Integrating the science and art of Nurse Coaching

- Professional trends and issues related to Nurse Coaching

- The Nurse Coach role in national and global healthcare transformation

- Nursing theories and other theories frequently used in professional Nurse Coaching practice

- Interventions frequently used in professional Nurse Coaching practice

- Glossary of terms related to professional Nurse Coaching practice

NOTE

1. In 2010 the National Consortium for the Credentialing of Health and Wellness Coaches (NCCHWC) convened to develop consensus around health and wellness coaching (NCCHWC, 2010; 2011; Wolever & Eisenberg, 2011). Over 80 individuals and organizations representing coaching, health care, and wellness discussed the development of credentialing standards for health and wellness coaching, and the need to integrate coaching skills into the health professions. (See NCCHWC, 2010; 2011). Retrieved from http://www.wellcoaches.com/images/pdf/progressreport-nationalteam-jul-2011.pdf).

Members from the Professional Nurse Coaching Workgroup (PNCW), the American Holistic Nurses Certification Corporation (AHNCC), and the American Holistic Nurses Association (AHNA) attended the meeting. Collaboration continues between the PNCW, nursing and the National Consortium. All PNCW members currently serve on different NCCHWC committees.

Overview of Content

✦ Foundational Professional Nursing Documents That Guide Professional Nurse Coaching Practice

Nurse Coaches are guided in their thinking and decision-making by three professional resources. *Nursing: Scope and Standards of Practice,* 2nd Edition (ANA, 2010a) outlines the expectations of the professional role of registered nurses. It provides the Scope of Practice for all registered nurses and the Standards of Professional Nursing Practice and their accompanying competencies. *Code of Ethics for Nurses with Interpretive Statements* (ANA, 2001) lists the nine provisions that establish the ethical framework for registered nurses across all roles, levels, and settings. *Nursing's Social Policy Statement: The Essence of Professional Practice* (ANA, 2010b) conceptualizes nursing practice, describes the social context of nursing, articulates professional nursing's social contract with society, and provides the definition of nursing.

[Note: The reader is referred to Appendix A for Background, Appendix B for the American Holistic Nurses Credentialing Corporation (AHNCC) Nurse Coach Certification Process, and Appendix C for the Nurse Coach Role in National and Global Healthcare Transformation as related to The Art and Science of Nurse Coaching: The Provider's Guide to Coaching Scope and Competencies.]

Additional Resources

The Art and Science of Nurse Coaching incorporates coaching standards and competencies of the International Coaching Federation (ICF) (2011a). The ICF, with more than 18,000 members in 100 countries (ICF, 2011b), provides independent certification for coaches. ICF certification is a certification process open to all who complete approved coach training, pass an oral and written examination, and meet practice hours requirements. It does not certify any specialties. It does, however, provide a rich resource with an established code of ethics (ICF, 2011c), body of research data, and delineation of practices essential to coaching.

Nurse Coaches practicing in a nursing specialty are also guided by the nursing specialty standards and related documents.

Audience for the Publication

Registered nurses in every role and setting constitute the primary audience of this professional resource. Nurse administrators, organizations and agencies (hospitals, community care centers, long term care facilities) legislators, regulators, legal counsel, and the judiciary system also will benefit from referencing this resource as the dynamic healthcare landscape changes. Those individuals, families, communities, and populations using healthcare and nursing services can use this document to better understand what constitutes professional Nurse Coaching by registered nurses.

Professional Nurse Coach Role: Definition and Scope of Practice

In this section the definition of the professional Nurse Coach role, the contexts of Nurse Coaching, and a detailed description of the practice will be found. In addition are the underlying tenets of practice and the organizing framework based on *Nursing: Scope and Standards of Practice*, 2nd Edition. (ANA, 2010a). *[Note: The word "client" is interchangeable with the word "patient" throughout this document.]*

Definition of Professional Nurse Coach and Professional Nurse Coaching

The professional Nurse Coach is a registered nurse who integrates coaching competencies into any setting or specialty area of practice to facilitate a process of change or development that assists individuals or groups to realize their potential. The change process is grounded in an awareness that effective change evolves from within before it can be manifested and maintained externally. The Nurse Coach works with the whole person, using principles and modalities that integrate body-mind-emotion-spirit-environment.

Professional Nurse Coaching is a skilled, purposeful, results-oriented, and structured relationship-centered interaction with clients provided by registered nurses for the purpose of promoting achievement of client goals. Achievement of client goals is accomplished by first establishing a co-creative partnership with the client where the client is the expert and then by identifying the client's priorities and areas for change. Goals originate from clarifying and identifying the client's agenda.

Professional Nurse Coaching Scope of Practice

The Art and Science of Nurse Coaching describes a competent level of professional Nurse Coaching practice and performance common to all Nurse Coaches. Effective Nurse Coaching interactions involve the ability to develop a coaching partnership, to create a safe space, and to be sensitive to client issues of trust and vulnerability (Schaub & Schaub, 2013; Schaub & Schaub, 2009) as a basis for further exploration, self-discovery and action planning related to desired outcomes. It builds on the client's strengths rather than attempting to "fix" weaknesses. Coaching interactions are based on research findings related to positive psychology (Seligman, 1990; Csikszentmihalyi, 1990) and learned optimism (Seligman, 1990) as it relates to transformational change (Prochaska, et.al., 1995).

The Nurse Coach must be able to explore client readiness for coaching, structure a coaching session, facilitate achievement of the client's desired goals, and co-create a means of determining and evaluating desired outcomes and goals (Hess, Bark, & Southard, 2010). Nurse Coaching is grounded in the principles and core values of professional nursing.

Professional Nurse Coaching practice:

- Incorporates both the *science* (critical thinking, use of evidence/ research/ theory [e.g., nursing theories, change theory including appreciative inquiry and motivational interviewing, coherence theory, resilience, complexity science, etc.] and *art* [e.g., intuition, creativity, presence, self-awareness assessment tools and practices, mindfulness, imagery, relaxation, music, etc.]).

- Includes the values and ethics of holism, caring, moral insight, dignity, integrity, competence, responsibility, accountability, and legality that underlie professional nursing.

- Incorporates culturally relevant philosophies and paradigms in a manner that promotes the achievement of client-centered goals.

- Recognizes that coaching interventions, inherent client characteristics, cultural norms, and policies and systems influence client outcomes.

- Honors the relationship between the client's internal and external environment in order to achieve optimal outcomes.

- Partners with the client to identify the client's agenda relative to achievement of the client's goals.

- Creates a safe environment for relationship-centered coaching that includes empathy, warmth, caring, compassion, authenticity, respect, trust, and humor if appropriate.

- Integrates professional nursing and coaching competencies to foster the achievement of client goals.

- Recognizes that self-development (e.g., self-reflection, self-assessment, and self-care) is necessary to provide effective Nurse Coaching services.

- Values self in professional Nurse Coaching practice.

Description and Scope of Professional Nurse Coaching Practice

Nurse Coaches work in all areas of nursing practice and interact with individuals and with groups. Nurse Coaches are staff nurses, ambulatory care nurses, case managers, advanced practice nurses, nursing faculty, nurse researchers, educators, administrators, or nurse entrepreneurs. Nurse Coaches may practice in a specialty area such as diabetes education, cardiac rehabilitation, or end-of-life care.

Nurse Coaches may focus on health and wellness coaching, executive coaching, faculty development coaching, managerial coaching, business coaching, or life coaching. The extent to which registered nurses engage in the Nurse Coach role is dependent on coach specific education, training, experience, position, and the population they serve. The Nurse Coaching competencies are applicable to all areas of professional Nurse Coaching practice.

Development and Function of Professional Nurse Coaching Competencies

The professional Nurse Coaching competencies are authoritative statements of the duties that all Nurse Coaches are expected to perform competently, regardless of setting or specialization. The list of competencies is not exhaustive. The contents of this document will be expanded and revised through time, as new and broader patterns of the Nurse Coach role are developed and accepted by the nursing profession. The Nurse Coach role, scope of practice, tenets, and competencies are subject to formal periodic review and revision.

Application of the competencies is dependent on context. Whether the specifics of each competency apply depends upon the purpose of the coaching interaction. With increased mastery of competencies the nurse is better able to coach the client.

✗ The Nursing Process

The nursing process involves six focal areas: assessment, diagnosis, outcomes identification, planning, implementation, and evaluation. These six areas are conceptualized as bi-directional feedback loops from each component (ANA, 2010a). The Nurse Coach uses caring as the essence of professional Nurse Coaching practice (ANA, 2010a) and recognizes the transpersonal dimension of the caring-healing relationship between nurse and client. (Dossey, 2013; Watson, 2007). The Nurse Coach uses the nurse caring process (Potter & Frisch, 2013) with a shift in terminology and meaning to understand and incorporate the client's subjective experience: from *assessment* to establishing a relationship and identifying readiness for change and the resources available to the client for change; from nursing *diagnosis* to identifying opportunities and issues; from *outcomes identification* to having the client set the agenda for achievement of the client's goals; from *planning* to creating the structure of the coaching interaction; from *implementation* to empowering the client to reach goals; and from *evaluation* to assisting the client to determine the extent to which goals were achieved. The Nurse Coach understands that growth and improved health, wholeness, and well-being are the result of an ongoing journey that is ever expanding.

✗ The Nurse Coaching Process

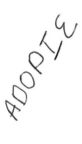

- **Establishing Relationship and Identifying Readiness for Change** (**Assessment**): The Nurse Coach begins by becoming fully present with self and client before initiating the coaching interaction. Cultivating and establishing relationship with the client is a priority for effective coaching. Nurse Coaching is a relationship-centered caring process. Assessment involves identifying the client's strengths, what the client wants to change, and assisting the client to determine his/her readiness for change. Assessment is dynamic and ongoing.

- **Identifying Opportunities, Issues, and Concerns (Diagnosis**): The Nurse Coach, in partnership with the client, identifies opportunities and issues related to growth, overall health, wholeness, and well-being. Opportunities for celebrating well-being are explored. The Nurse Coach understands that acknowledgment promotes and reinforces previous successes and serves to enhance further achievements. *Note: There is no attempt or need to assign labels or to establish a diagnosis* *when coaching. Instead the Nurse Coach is open to multiple interpretations of an unfolding interaction.*

- **Establishing Client-Centered Goals (Outcomes identification):** The Nurse Coach employs an overall approach to each coaching interaction that is designed to facilitate achievement of client goals and desired results.

- **Creating the Structure of the Coaching Interaction (Planning):** The Nurse Coach may structure the coaching interaction with a coaching agreement that identifies specific parameters of the coaching relationship, including coach and client responsibilities and action plans.

- **Empowering and Motivating Clients to Reach Goals (Implementation):** The Nurse Coach employs effective communication skills such as deep listening, powerful questioning, and directed dialogue as key components of the coaching interaction. In partnership with the client, the Nurse Coach facilitates learning and results by co-creating awareness, designing actions, setting goals, planning, and addressing progress and accountability. The Nurse Coach skillfully chooses interventions based on the client's statements and actions, and interacts with intention and curiosity in a manner that assists the client toward achievement of the client's goals. The Nurse Coach effectively uses her/his nursing knowledge and a variety of skills acquired with additional coach training.

- **Assisting Client to Determine the Extent to which Goals were Achieved (Evaluation):** The Nurse Coach is aware that evaluation of coaching (the nursing intervention) is done primarily by the client and is based on the client's perception of success and achievement of client-centered goals. The nurse partners with the client to evaluate progress toward goals.

Tenets and Characteristics of Professional Nurse Coaching Practice

The following professional Nurse Coaching tenets are embedded in every competency in this document and are reflected in professional Nurse Coaching practice.

1. The Nurse Coach's practice is individualized for the client.

The Nurse Coach encourages growth, wholeness, and well-being of the client according to the client's values and beliefs, and believes that every client is creative, resourceful, and whole. A *client* is defined as the person, patient, family member, community, group, or population. There is unity, totality, and connectedness of everyone and everything: human beings are unique and inherently good. People are able to find meaning and purpose in life experiences. All people have an innate power and capacity for the achievement of well-being. People are the recipients of Nurse Coaching services.

2. The Nurse Coach establishes a coaching relationship with the client.

The Nurse Coach establishes a coaching relationship as foundational to the success of a coaching interaction. It is a relationship where the complexity of human experiences is valued. The Nurse Coach demonstrates unconditional positive regard for clients and accepts them where they are. Within the Nurse Coach–client relationship, it is understood that change is best achieved when aligned with the client's goals and desires and readiness for change.

3. Human caring is central to professional Nurse Coaching practice.

Human caring is the moral ideal of nursing in which the nurse brings one's entire self into a relationship with the whole self of the client in order to protect the client's vulnerability, preserve her or his humanity and dignity, and reinforce the meaning and experience of oneness and unity.

4. The Nurse Coach uses the Nurse Coaching process to guide nurse-client coaching interactions.

The Nurse Coaching process is a systematic and skilled process that incorporates approaches to nursing practice and the coaching process that are holistic, integrative, and integral. The nursing process is expanded and reinterpreted to include widely used nursing theories and evidence-based behavioral change theories and frameworks that redefine established concepts and terms. The Nurse Coach understands and adheres to professional and ethical standards that include providing respectful, compassionate, and culturally relevant integrative nursing care to all persons.

5. **The Nurse Coach recognizes the link between the internal and external environment of self and the client.**

Each component influences growth, health, optimal functioning, and well-being.

Healthy Environments (Internal and External) for Professional Nurse Coaching Practice

The environment is the context within which all living systems participate and interact, including the physical body and its habitat along with cultural, psychological, social, and historical influences. It includes both the external physical space and the person's internal physical, mental, emotional, social, and spiritual experience. Well-being is possible for all. Illness and/or imbalance provide opportunities for learning and movement toward change to enhance well-being (AHNA/ANA, 2013).

ANA Standards as Organizing Framework for Professional Nurse Coaching Practice

The six Standards of Practice and ten Standards of Professional Performance in *Nursing: Scope and Standards of Practice*, 2nd Edition (ANA, 2010a) provide the organizing framework for *The Art and Science of Nurse Coaching*. Competencies specific to the professional Nurse Coach role that are described in this document (starting on page 27) are linked to those standards, which are reproduced in the following table for the convenience of the reader.

Standards of Practice	Standards of Professional Practice
The Standards of Practice describe a competent level of nursing care as demonstrated by the critical thinking model known as the nursing process. The nursing process includes the components of assessment, diagnosis, outcomes identification, planning, implementation, and evaluation. Accordingly, the nursing process encompasses significant actions taken by registered nurses and forms the foundation of the nurse's decision-making.	The Standards of Professional Performance describe a competent level of behavior in the professional role, including activities related to ethics, education, evidence-based practice and research, quality of practice, communication, leadership, collaboration, professional practice evaluation, resource utilization, and environmental health.
Standard 1. Assessment The registered nurse collects comprehensive data pertinent to the healthcare consumer's health and/or the situation.	All registered nurses are expected to engage in professional role activities, including leadership, appropriate to their education and position. Registered nurses are accountable for their professional actions to themselves, their healthcare consumers, their peers, and ultimately to society.
Standard 2. Diagnosis The registered nurse analyzes the assessment data to determine the diagnoses or the issues.	**Standard 7. Ethics** The registered nurse practices ethically.
Standard 3. Outcomes Identification The registered nurse identifies expected outcomes for a plan individualized to the healthcare consumer or the situation.	**Standard 8. Education** The registered nurse attains knowledge and competence that reflects current nursing practice.
Standard 4. Planning The registered nurse develops a plan that prescribes strategies and alternatives to attain expected outcomes.	**Standard 9. Evidence-Based Practice and Research** The registered nurse integrates evidence and research findings into practice.
Standard 5. Implementation The registered nurse implements the identified plan.	**Standard 10. Quality of Practice** The registered nurse contributes to quality nursing practice.
Standard 6. Evaluation The registered nurse evaluates progress toward attainment of outcomes.	**Standard 11. Communication** The registered nurse communicates effectively in a variety of formats in all areas of practice.
	Standard 12. Leadership The registered nurse demonstrates leadership in the professional practice setting and the profession.
	Standard 13. Collaboration The registered nurse collaborates with healthcare consumer, family, and others in the conduct of nursing practice.

Standards of Practice	Standards of Professional Practice
	Standard 14. Professional Practice Evaluation The registered nurse evaluates her or his own nursing practice in relation to professional practice standards and guidelines, relevant statutes, and regulations.
	Standard 15. Resource Utilization The registered nurse utilizes appropriate resources to plan and provide nursing services that are safe, effective, and financially responsible.
	Standard 16. Environmental Health The registered nurse practices in an environmentally safe and healthy manner.

Professional Competence in Nurse Coaching Practice

Professional Nurse Coaching competence can be taught, defined, measured, and evaluated. There is no single method of evaluation or tool that can guarantee competence. Competence is dynamic and situational and is recognized as an ongoing process resulting in appropriate outcome/s. The context of a coaching relationship/coaching interaction determines what competencies are necessary. Assurance of competence is the shared responsibility of individual nurses, professional nursing organizations, credentialing and certification entities, and other key stakeholders.

Definitions and Concepts Related to Professional Nurse Coaching Competence

The following ideas are central to the discussion of Nurse Coaching competence:

- A Nurse Coach who demonstrates competence (per the competencies in this document) is performing at an expected level.

- A Nurse Coach competency is an expected level of performance that integrates knowledge, skills, abilities, and judgment.

- A Nurse Coach integrates knowledge, skills, abilities, and judgment in formal, informal, and reflective learning experiences.

- A Nurse Coach has integrity.

- A Nurse Coach is aware of her/his own strengths and weaknesses, has positive self-regard, and is open to feedback.

- A Nurse Coach values and uses intuitive knowing.

- Nurse Coaching involves emotional, moral, and spiritual intelligence.

- Nurse Coaching demonstrates an understanding of science and humanities, professional standards of practice, coaching competencies, insights gained from experiences, personal strengths, resources, and capabilities, and leadership performance.

- Nurse Coaching includes psychomotor, communication, interpersonal, and environmental skills.

- Nurse Coaching judgment includes critical thinking, problem-solving, ethical reasoning, decision-making, and clinical leadership.

- Nurse Coach learning may occur in academic settings, professional practice environments, structured certificate programs, and online educational offerings.

- Nurse Coach reflective learning is recurrent thoughtful self-assessment, analysis, and synthesis of strengths and opportunities for improvement.

Competence and Competency in Professional Nurse Coaching Practice

The competent Nurse Coach considers the person, family, and/or group being coached and the setting and available resources. The Nurse Coach considers factors that either enhance or detract from the ability to conduct a coaching session or coaching interaction. The Nurse Coach addresses barriers that constrain competent practice. The ability to perform at the expected level requires lifelong learning and self-development (self-reflection, self-assessment, self-evaluation, and self-care). Nurse Coaches continually assess and reassess their competencies and identify areas where new knowledge, skills, integral learning experiences, and self-development can enhance personal and professional self-development.

Evaluating Competence

Competence is evaluated using measurement tools that capture qualitative and quantitative data about the Nurse Coach's basic knowledge and performance. However, no single tool or method can guarantee competence.

Professional Nurse Coaching Practice Today

Statistical Snapshot

There are 3.1 million nurses in the United States (ANA, 2010a; AACN, 2011). It is the largest segment of the nation's healthcare workforce. A major shift is underway in the United States to move from a disease-based model of care to a health and wellness promotion model. New national prevention strategies are being considered and implemented. Currently there are 17.6 millions nurses and midwives engaged in providing healthcare around the world (WHO, 2009).

The role of the Nurse Coach is fundamental to professional nursing (Schaub, Luck & Dossey, 2013). The Nurse Coach role has roots in social sciences, holism, and nursing theory. Nurse coaching competencies are based in nursing, behavioral science, and health promotion theories and research. Development of professional Nurse Coaching skills, which integrate basic coaching skills with the unique dimensions that shape nursing practice, is not typically included in the curriculums of nursing educational programs. The focused preparation of Nurse Coaches is integral to ensuring these services are available to patients.

Health and wellness coaches without a professional health background have emerged. In 2010 the National Consortium for the Credentialing of Health and Wellness Coaches (NCCHWC) convened to develop consensus around health and wellness coaching (National Consortium for the Credentialing of Health and Wellness Coaches Progress Report July, 2011; Wolever & Eisenberg, 2011). Over 80 individuals and organizations representing coaching, health care, and wellness discussed the development of credentialing standards for health and wellness coaching, and the need to integrate coaching competencies into the health professions.

It is an important time for the nursing profession to expand its visibility by embracing the professional Nurse Coach role and the emerging coaching paradigm. With the national focus on prevention and wellness promotion, it is essential for nursing to have an increased presence in health and wellness efforts designed to improve health outcomes and reduce health costs for individuals, employers, insurance companies, and the nation.

Nurse Coaches must assume a significant leadership role in these efforts. It is critical that available professional nurse resources be maximized to reduce the prevalence and severity of chronic illness. Nurse Coaches are equipped to implement health-promoting strategies with clients, supporting behavioral and lifestyle changes to enhance growth, overall health and well-being.

The Art and Science of Nurse Coaching describes the role of the Nurse Coach. It will assist nurses as they assume the position of Nurse Coach in hospitals, clinics, communities, and in private professional nurse practices. It will serve as a guide in the development of Nurse Coach educational programs. Reimbursement is also needed for Nurse Coaching that is already being provided in wellness promotion programs that are included within managed care contracts that have been implemented into new Medicare programs.

Roots of Professional Nurse Coaching

Florence Nightingale (1820–1910)—the foundational philosopher of modern nursing—established nursing practice that could be measured by evaluating outcomes. She advocated, identified, and focused on factors that promote health recognized today as environmental and social determinants of health—the same factors that Nurse Coaches now promote to achieve optimal health and well-being (Dossey, 2013; Dossey, 2010; Dossey, Selanders, Beck, & Attewell, 2005; Nightingale, 1859, 1860, 1893). Nightingale emphasized the necessity for nursing to be a profession, and that nurses must be educated, and not "trained." She established the imperative of evidence-based practice, a nursing standard now widely known to be as important as she had known it to be. Nightingale was the first recognized nurse theorist—a clinical educator, scientist, statistician, environmentalist, policy maker, social activist, facilitator, communicator, and visionary. Her contributions to nursing theory, research, statistics, public health, healthcare reform, and Nurse Coaching are foundational and inspirational. In 1893 Nightingale wrote:

..."In the future which I shall not see, for I am old, may a better way be opened! May the methods by which every infant, every human being will have the best chance at health—the methods by which every sick person will have the best chance at recovery, be learned and practiced. Hospitals are only an intermediate stage of civilization, never intended, at all events, to take in the whole sick population.

May we hope that, when we are all dead and gone, leaders will arise who have been personally experienced in the hard, practical work, the difficulties, and the joys of organizing nursing reforms, and who will lead far beyond anything we have done..."

Nightingale left 21st-century nurses with a call. Nurse Coaches bring an integrative, holistic perspective to coaching (Dossey, 2013; Dossey, 2010; Hess et al., 2010). Nurse theorists and scholars have created models for working with the whole person that incorporate the biological, psychological, social/cultural, environmental, and transpersonal and energetic components of individuals. Integral perspectives allow for openness and "not knowing" (Dossey, 2009) – a way to where new knowledge resides. Erickson views this broad outlook as "integrative knowing," "a way to bring together "multiple ways-of-knowing, integrating and creating new knowledge" (Erickson, 2010, p. 65). Some Nurse Coaches utilize a holistic, integral model of coaching as a way to frame coaching interactions (Bark, 2011; Bark Coaching Institute, n.d.; Integrative Nurse Coach Certificate Program, n.d.).

Professional Nurse Coaching Research and Evidence-Based Practice

Professional Nurse Coaching research is relevant to learning, documenting, and comprehending the science and art of Nurse Coaching. To increase the understanding of professional Nurse Coaching practice and to enhance the evidence-base, research may include descriptive, explanatory and exploratory designs. This may be accomplished by using qualitative, quantitative, mixed methods or other approaches. Professional Nurse Coaching research is needed to further the understanding of the Nurse Coach–client relationship. This will support identifying the factors that contribute to increased client efficacy and ability to successfully achieve the changes that enhance life satisfaction, growth, health, and well-being.

Evidence-based practice is the conscientious use of the best available evidence combined with clinician's expertise and judgment, and patient's preferences and values to arrive at the best decisions leading to quality outcomes (Baldwin, Schultz, Melynk, & Rycoft-Malone, 2013). Nurse Coaches honor the individual's subjective health experiences, health beliefs, and values. Nurse Coaches develop therapeutic partnerships with individuals, families, and communities that are grounded in nursing knowledge, theories, research expertise, intuition, and creativity. Nurse researchers are encouraged to design Nurse Coaching research studies that incorporate theories, conceptual frameworks, and a paradigm that strengthens the understanding of the whole person (Zahourek, 2013.)

Professional Nurse Coaching research and evidence-based practice is growing. Numerous articles in scholarly nursing journals referring to Nurse Coaching have been published (Hess & Dossey, in press). As the national focus continues to move from disease care to health promotion and wellness, additional research is needed.

Professional Nurse Coaching in Advocacy and Society

Chronic disease and stress related illnesses are increasing. The fast pace of daily life, lack of exercise, poor food choices, and environmental risk factors are frequently implicated. Nurse Coaching is critical to assisting individuals, families, and groups to make the changes that foster self-awareness and promote healthier lifestyles.

Nurse Coaches have the skills and knowledge to empower individuals to make beneficial changes. Furthermore, Nurse Coaches have the ability to help transform the health of our nation and our world as they engage in interprofessional conversations and partnerships to facilitate the changes that lead to improved health and well-being.

Progression of Professional Nurse Coaching Curriculum Development, Nurse Coaching Certificate Programs, and Professional Nurse Coaching Certification

As the role of the Nurse Coach has evolved, it is apparent that the term *coach* is loosely defined and often confused with the role of preceptor, mentor, counselor, navigator, or educator. Although growing in popularity, the role of the Nurse Coach has not been clearly defined. *The Art and Science of Nurse Coaching* addresses the need to clearly define the role of the Nurse Coach and provides a guide for nurses across all nursing specialties, for Nurse Coach curriculum development, for Nurse Coach certificate programs, and for Nurse Coach certification.

Health and wellness programs, health maintenance organizations, health insurance companies, and agencies that provide case management services are increasingly employing nurses as coaches to assist individuals in achieving improved health outcomes. Many nurses in hospitals and community agencies have added coaching skills to their nursing practice as a new strategy or intervention to assist patients. Some nurses who professionally pursue such coaching have created successful and thriving businesses providing coach training and coaching services to private clients, groups, and organizations. These early indicators of the importance and impact of nurses as professional coaches emphasize the urgency in formally defining the role, scope of practice, and competencies of the Nurse Coach.

In the 1950s, nursing theorists Hildegard Peplau and Dorothea Orem introduced several concepts and practices that are now seen as important elements of professional Nurse Coaching practice.

Peplau (1952) described the nurse's task as recognizing and mobilizing the person's innate capacity for self-healing and growth. Her perspective originated in a belief that every individual is a unique being with the capacity to learn, develop, and change. She saw the role of the nurse as collaborating and partnering with the client to establish a relationship that would assist the client to realize these potentials. She wrote of the importance of the nurse's self-awareness and self-knowledge in order that this process would occur free of the nurse's needs and agendas. Peplau wrote of clarifying, listening, accepting and interpreting what the client shared in the interpersonal relationship. As part of the resolution process, the nurse would assist the client in establishing new goals, if desired.

Orem (1971) first wrote of her self-care model of nursing in 1953. Her work emerged from a philosophy of health as a state of wholeness. She identified self-care as a key element in maintaining human structure and functioning throughout the lifecycle. The nurse works with clients in helping to identify their self-care deficits. The nurse then helps the client to overcome the deficits by addressing the client's capacity and motivation to do so. Orem recognized that taking responsibility for self-care was a role change for the client. She wrote of the importance of the client-nurse relationship as being instrumental in supporting a process of change.

Patricia Benner (1985), the prominent nurse leader, theorist, and author of the nursing textbook *From Novice to Expert* (Benner, 1984) used the term *nurse coach* nearly 30 years ago to describe the patient–nurse partnership and a conceptual framework based on social support theory. In her model, the nurse responds to and interacts with the client to create joint decision-making regarding goals and methods to achieve goals. This coaching or partnering process involves a nursing perspective that includes holism and self-care and guides Nurse Coaches in the mobilization of inner resources and inner wisdom.

Schenk (2002) described the nurse coach as a healthcare resource for this millennium. Southard (2003) developed a health coach integrative model of care for nurses with accompanying standards of practice based on the core values of holistic nursing. Hayes and Kalmakis (2007) described coaching as a significant strategy available to nurse practitioners to promote health and wellness by inviting the active participation of the individual receiving healthcare services. In 2008 Watson developed the Caring Science Caritas Coaching Education Program (CCEP) (Watson Caring Science Institute, n.d.). Watson's Caritas Coaching Program focuses on intelligent heart-centered approaches to health care by translating and sustaining the ethic, philosophy, theory, and practice of the Science of Human Caring into systems and society (Watson Caring Science Institute, n.d.).

In 2009, the International Council of Nurses (ICN), a federation of more than 130 national nursing organization and representing millions of nurses worldwide, partnered with the Honor Society of Nursing, Sigma Theta Tau International (STTI), representing over 125,000 nurses worldwide, and published *Coaching in Nursing* (Donner & Wheeler, 2009) to support this direction for professional development of nurses.

McNally and Cunningham (2010) developed a coaching model that focuses on helping nurse leaders conduct coaching conversations for development of coaching cultures in the workplace. Bark (2011) developed an integral model of coaching based on structures of consciousness and integral theory that has been taught and used by many nurses in professional nursing practice. Bark's coaching model provides a multidimensional foundation and methods for coaching and coach training (Bark Coaching Institute, n.d.). Dossey, Luck, and Schaub developed the Integrative Nurse Coach Certificate Program (INCCP) based on integral theory, the vulnerability model, and the integrative functional health model, as well as other recognized coaching theories and competencies. Nurses develop coaching skills to assist clients in the achievement of health and wellness goals and to navigate the complex world of medical care (Integrative Nurse Coach Certificate Program, n.d.).

IOM Influences on Professional Nurse Coaching Practice and Leadership

Undertaking a two-year study started in 2008, the Robert Wood Johnson Foundation (RWJF) and the Institute of Medicine (IOM) partnered to assess the future of the nursing profession. The intention was to determine ways to transform the profession of nursing. The outcome of this process was a report that makes recommendations for an action-oriented blueprint for the future of nursing.

The IOM report *The Future of Nursing* (2010) developed four key messages:

- Nurses should practice to the full extent of their education and training.

- Nurses should achieve higher levels of education and training through an improved education system that promotes seamless academic progression.

- Nurses should be full partners, with physicians and other healthcare professionals, in redesigning health care in the United States.

- Effective workforce planning and policy making require better data collection and information infrastructure.

As the United States transforms its healthcare system, professional Nurse Coaches are emerging as leaders who play a fundamental role in informing the government, regulatory agencies, businesses, and organizations about professional Nurse Coaching practice.

Integrating the Science and Art of Nurse Coaching

Nurse Coaching Core Values

Nurse Coaches understand that the professional Nurse Coach role, scope of practice, and competencies are linked to each of the ANA six Standards of Practice and ten Standards of Professional Performance (ANA, 2010a). The professional Nurse Coach role is based upon the following five core values: (1) Nurse Coach Philosophy, Theories, Ethics; (2) Nurse Coaching Process; (3) Nurse Coach Communication, Coaching Environment; (4) Nurse Coach Education, Research, Leadership; and (5) Nurse Coach Self-Development (Self-Reflection, Self-Assessment, Self-Evaluation, Self-Care).

These core values and the specific Nurse Coaching competencies—which are aligned with *Nursing: Scope and Standards of Practice*, 2nd Edition (ANA, 2010a) and *Holistic Nursing: Scope and Standards*, 2nd Edition. (AHNA & ANA, 2013)—are the foundation for curriculum development, while *Professional Nurse Coach Core Curriculum* (Dossey & Hess, in press), and the nationally recognized American Holistic Nurses Credentialing Corporation (AHNCC) Nurse Coach Certification process (see Appendix B). Nurse Coaches understand that professional Nurse Coaching practice is defined by these core values and competencies. Nurse Coaching enhances foundational professional nursing skills that are acquired by additional training.

The Science of Nurse Coaching

Nurse Coaches incorporate approaches to nursing practice that are holistic, integrative, and integral and which include the work of numerous nurse scholars. Nurse Coaching is a systematic and skilled process grounded in scholarly evidenced-based professional nursing practice. (Appendix C discusses nursing and other related theories and concepts commonly utilized in professional Nurse Coaching practice.)

The Art of Nurse Coaching

The nurse caring process guides the establishment of core values and competencies of professional Nurse Coaching practice, whether used with individuals, families, groups, or communities. At the heart of Nurse Coaching is growth of the body-mind-spirit system on various levels. The quality of human caring is central in the Nurse Coach–client relationship. The nurse brings her/his self into the coaching relationship with the whole self of the patient/client. This relationship provides the client with a safe environment in which to express their feelings, goals, hopes, dreams, and share their vulnerability, pain, and suffering.

This relationship allows a flow of energy in the body-mind-spirit system of each that may be manifested as creativity, coherence, resilience, or anxiety, fear and frustration (Koerner, 2011). The Nurse Coach holds the container for what needs to be expressed. In the coaching relationship there may be various shifts in consciousness, intrapersonal dynamics, interpersonal relationships, and expressions of the lived experiences of connection, unity, and oneness with the larger environment, cosmos, or Spirit, however defined. Ideally Nurse Coaches embody the following qualities (Dossey, Luck, & Schaub, 2013):

- Development of integrative, integral, and holistic perspectives that include a bio-psycho-social-spiritual-cultural-environmental model of the person

- Recognition that self-healing is an on-going process and necessitates intentionality

- Willingness to model self-development (self-reflection, self-assessments, self-evaluation, self-care)

- Willingness to identify creative and self-defeating patterns in self

- Willingness to take responsibility for inner reactions to clients and situations

- Commitment to maintain a sense of presence, authenticity, and self-awareness in nursing practice

- Cultivation of a capacity for deep listening, mindful presence, and not-knowing

- Respect and love for the humanness of clients

- Commitment to creativity and innovation

- Willingness to bear witness to a client's pain and suffering

- Willingness to believe that change is possible for all

- Commitment to life-long personal self-development and learning

In professional Nurse Coaching practice the nurse attends to the client's subjective experiences and the client's internal frame of reference. The Nurse Coach views clients as resourceful individuals with inherent answers and wisdom. The client chooses the topics for coaching and determines the direction of the coaching session. The nurse sets aside the expert role. There is no predetermined information or education to be offered, and there are no predetermined objectives or outcomes identified.

Professional Nurse Coaching recognizes and supports the client's current way of being as the client evolves towards desired changes and goals. The Nurse Coach spends time with the client in discovery and only moves into the nurse expert role, when indicated, to assist the client. The Nurse Coach remembers that "less is more" when it comes to teaching or advising. What needs to be shared emerges as the nurse "walks with the client" through the discovery process.

The Nurse Coach is present, curious, attentive to the present moment, and thus open to what emerges, free of any predetermined idea of what needs to be "fixed" in the client. The Nurse Coach listens carefully and attentively to the thread of a client's story, perspectives, and reality while engaging in a skillful and free-flowing process of discovery. The Nurse Coach trusts her/his intuition regarding what to say next, and is not thinking about the next question. By skillfully using the "power of the pause," the Nurse Coach communicates being comfortable with silence and is then able to be totally present and open to what the client is expressing.

Professional Nurse Coaching Societal and Ethical Dimensions

Nurses are bound by a professional code of ethics (ANA, 2001). At the heart of nursing's social contract with society is self-regulation by the nursing profession that assures quality performance. Nurses are responsive to the changing needs of society regarding the expansion of theoretical and scientific parameters related to human flourishing, health promotion and disease prevention. Nurse Coaches are accountable for their performance. They engage in quality reviews to further refine their professional knowledge, competence, communication, and leadership.

Nurse Coaches work independently as well as collaboratively to leverage overlapping skills that complement individual efforts (ANA, 2010a). Recognizing the expertise of interprofessional colleagues, they make referrals when appropriate. This may entail shared responsibilities with a common focus on clients' reaching their highest potential. Nurse Coaches recognize their constantly changing professional practice boundaries. Nurse Coaches frequently evaluate safety, effectiveness, and costs related to the services they provide. They are committed to lifelong learning.

Caring and Professional Nurse Coach Practice

Caring is the essence of nursing and central to the professional Nurse Coach role. Human caring is the moral ideal of nursing in which the nurse brings one's entire self into a relationship with the whole self of the client in order to protect the client's vulnerability, preserve her or his humanity and dignity, and reinforce the meaning and experience of oneness and unity. Nurse Coaches recognize the transpersonal caring-healing process (Dossey, 2013; Watson,

2007) that involves temporarily transcending or moving beyond one's usual identification with the limited biological, historical, cultural, and personal self; this occurs at the deepest and most profound levels of human experience possible. Transpersonal refers to that which transcends the limits and boundaries of individual ego identities and possibilities to include acknowledgment and appreciation of something greater.

Continued Commitment to Professional Nurse Coaching

Nurse Coaches remain involved in continuous learning and self-development to enhance Nurse Coaching practice. Nurse Coaches may demonstrate commitment to their practices by their involvement in professional associations and community organizations, by acquiring additional education, or by other self-development activities (e.g. supervision, continuing education, reflection, self-assessment, lifestyle changes).

Nurse Coaches possess the knowledge, skills, and abilities to assist clients to achieve goals. Nurse Coaches facilitate changes that foster improved health and well-being for all regardless of cultural background, value system, religious belief, gender, sexual identity, or disability. Nurse Coaches believe that change is possible and are willing to hold that vision for all.

Professional Trends and Issues Related to Professional Nurse Coaching

It is estimated that 270 billion dollars a year is spent on disease management—on attempting to cure acute disease and treat chronic disease. According to the Centers for Disease Control and Prevention, in 2009, approximately 133 million Americans—nearly 1 in 2 adults—were living with at least one chronic illness and more than 70% of healthcare costs were due to preventable lifestyle-related diseases (Snyderman & Dinan, 2010). Currently, with eight out of ten people over 25 years of age overweight, and with childhood obesity spiraling out of control, the future burden on our health system and society provides an imperative to seek new directions to halt these trends (Luck, 2010). It is estimated that over ten years, $900 billion can be saved with lifestyle medicine (Hyman, Ornish, & Roizen, 2010). Lifestyle medicine involves engaging individuals in health promotion, assisting them to be proactive, participatory, and to partner with healthcare providers and others in creating new and sustainable health behaviors.

Chronic disease is now seen as a global epidemic and a driver for rising healthcare costs. The World Health Organization (WHO, 2011) reports that cardiovascular diseases (heart disease and strokes), cancers, diabetes and chronic lung disease are today the leading causes of disease burden and death worldwide. The four major causative chronic disease risk factors are tobacco use, unhealthy diet, lack of physical activity, and the harmful use of alcohol. Chronic illness is seen as a cause for early mortality that has now surpassed communicable disease.

The Patient Protection and Affordable Care Act, the Healthy People 2020 Initiative, and the National Prevention Strategy (see more below) have increased the national conversations related to new healthcare strategies.

Patient Protection and Affordable Care Act

On March 23, 2010, the Patient Protection and Affordable Care Act (PPACA) became law (HR3590) (The Patient Protection and Affordable Care Act, 2010). The language in the PPACA refers to partnerships in Section 4001 includes partnerships with a diverse group of licensed health professionals including practitioners of integrative health, preventive medicine, health coaching, public education, and more.

Healthy People 2020 Initiative

In December 2010 the Healthy People 2020 initiative (U.S. Department of Health and Human Services, n.d.) was announced. This initiative continues the work started in 2000 with the Healthy People 2010 initiative for improving the nation's health. The Healthy People 2020 initiative is the result of a multiyear process that reflects input from a diverse group of individuals and organizations. The leading health indicators are increased physical activity, overweight and obesity, tobacco use, substance abuse, responsible healthy sexual behavior, mental health, injury and violence, environmental quality, immunization, and access to health care. These health indicators were selected on the basis of their ability to motivate action, the availability of data to measure progress, and their importance as public health issues.

The vision, mission, and overarching goals provide structure and guidance for achieving the Healthy People 2020 objectives. While general in nature, they offer specific, important areas of emphasis where action must be taken if the United States is to achieve better health by the year 2020. Developed under the leadership of the Federal Interagency Workgroup (FIW), the Healthy People

2020 framework is the product of an exhaustive collaborative process among the U.S. Department of Health and Human Services (HHS) and other federal agencies, public stakeholders, and the advisory committee.

The Healthy People 2020 mission is to:

- Identify nationwide health improvement priorities.

- Increase public awareness and understanding of the determinants of health, disease, and disability and the opportunities for progress.

- Provide measurable objectives and goals that are applicable at the national, State, and local levels.

- Engage multiple sectors to take actions to strengthen policies and improve practices that are driven by the best available evidence and knowledge.

- Identify critical research, evaluation, and data collection needs.

The overall goals of Healthy People 2020 are to:

- Attain high-quality, longer lives free of preventable disease, disability, injury, and premature death.

- Achieve health equity, eliminate disparities, and improve the health of all groups.

- Create social and physical environments that promote good health for all.

- Promote quality of life, healthy development, and healthy behaviors across all life stages.

National Prevention Strategy

On June 16, 2011, the National Prevention, Health Promotion, and Public Health Council, including Surgeon General Regina Benjamin, MD, Department of Health and Human Services (HHS) Secretary Kathleen Sebelius, and others announced the release of the National Prevention and Health Promotion Strategy. Referred to subsequently as the National Prevention Strategy, it is a comprehensive plan that will help increase the number of Americans who are healthy at every stage of life (National Prevention Council, 2011, 2012). To stop disease before it starts and to create strategies for a healthy and fit nation, prevention must become part of daily life. The National Prevention Strategy recognizes that good health comes not just from receiving quality medical care, but also from clean air and water, safe worksites and healthy foods. The strategy was created through the PPACA and developed by the National Prevention Council, which is comprised of the heads of 17 Federal agencies that consulted with outside experts and stakeholders.

The National Prevention Strategy includes actions that public and private partners can take to help Americans stay healthy and fit and improve our nation's prosperity. The strategy outlines four strategic directions that, together, are fundamental to improving the nation's health:

- Building Healthy and Safe Community Environments: Prevention of disease starts in our communities and at home; not just in the doctor's office.

- Expanding Quality Preventive Services in Both Clinical and Community Settings: When people receive preventive care, such as immunizations and cancer screenings, they have better health and lower healthcare costs.

- Empowering People to Make Healthy Choices: When people have access to actionable and easy-to-understand information and resources, they are empowered to make healthier choices.

- Eliminating Health Disparities: By eliminating disparities in achieving and maintaining health, we can help improve quality of life for all Americans.

Other Federal Health and Wellness Programs

Specific actions are underway by the Obama Administration to implement programs to improve Americans' lives, including the America's Great Outdoors Initiative, the Neighborhood Revitalization Initiative, and Executive Order 13548 to make the federal government a model employer of persons with disabilities. Through these and other programs, the Obama Administration is working to ensure every American has the opportunity to live the healthiest life possible.

Nurse Coaches will be of assistance in achieving the goals of the Patient Protection and Affordable Care Act, the Healthy People 2020 Initiative, the National Prevention Strategy, and other programs being implemented to improve health and well-being for all.

Summary of the Scope of Nurse Coaching Practice

With a renewed focus on prevention and wellness promotion in healthcare reform, now is an important time for the nursing profession to expand its visibility in the emerging coaching paradigm. As various strategies gain momentum for the training of wellness coaches, Nurse Coaches are uniquely positioned to coach and engage individuals in the process of behavior change.

Professional Nurse Coach Practice and Performance Competencies

Professional Nurse Coach competencies are linked to each of the ANA six Standards of Practice and ten Standards of Professional Performance (ANA, 2010a). A description of the professional Nurse Coach role pertaining to each standard is provided followed by the specific Nurse Coach competencies related to that standard.

[Note: Professional Nurse Coach practice competencies include the ICF competencies.]

✗ Professional Nurse Coach Practice Competencies

ANA Standard 1. Assessment

The registered nurse collects comprehensive data pertinent to the healthcare consumer's health and/or the situation.

Professional Nurse Coach Role

Setting the foundation for coaching begins during the assessment phase of the coaching interaction. Assessment begins by becoming fully present with self and client before initiating the coaching interaction. Assessment proceeds to establishing a relationship with the client and access to the client's subjective experience/story and internal frame of reference through the cultivation and establishment of a relationship. The Nurse Coach determines if the client's concerns are appropriate for the coaching role. The Nurse Coach helps the client assess readiness and available resources for change. Assessment is dynamic and ongoing.

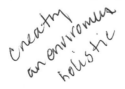

Professional Nurse Coach Competencies

The Nurse Coach:

1. Becomes fully present to self and client prior to collecting data pertinent to the coaching interaction.

2. Co-creates a relationship between the Nurse Coach and the client that promotes trust and intimacy.

3. Recognizes and respects the client as the authority on her or his own health and well-being.

4. Explores with the client why coaching is being considered at this time and what the client wants to address during the coaching interaction.

5. Ensures that the client sets the agenda for the coaching session and holds the client's agenda throughout the session.

X 6. Helps the client assess stage of readiness for change (pre-contemplation, contemplation, preparation, action, maintenance). List All

7. Incorporates various types of knowing, including intuition, and validates this intuitive knowledge with the client when appropriate.

8. Explores, through powerful questions and feedback, multiple sources of information to assist the client to become aware of areas for coaching.

X 9. Uses appropriate evidence-informed whole person assessment techniques and instruments, with the client's permission, and with appropriate training.

10. Determines the need for, and refers the client to, other professionals and services as appropriate.

X 11. Assesses if there is an effective working match between the coach and the prospective client.

12. Understands and effectively discusses with the client the ethical guidelines and specific parameters of the Nurse Coaching relationship (e.g., logistics, fees, scheduling).

X 13. Co-creates with the client an agreement that identifies the role of the Nurse Coach and the role of the client.

ANA Standard 2. Diagnosis

The registered nurse analyzes the assessment data to determine the diagnoses or the issues.

Professional Nurse Coach Role

The Nurse Coach and the client together explore assessment data to determine areas for change.

Professional Nurse Coach Competencies

The Nurse Coach:

1. Clarifies the client's issues and concerns and/or opportunities for change based on the whole person assessment data.

2. Confirms the client's issues and concerns and/or opportunities with the client.

3. Tracks the client's issues and concerns and/or opportunities in a manner that leads to identification of the client's goals that will be the focus of the coaching process.

ANA Standard 3. Outcomes Identification

The registered nurse identifies expected outcomes for a plan individualized to the healthcare consumer or the situation.

Professional Nurse Coach Role

The Nurse Coach assists the client to identify goals that will lead to the desired change. The Nurse Coach values the evolution and the process of change as it unfolds.

Professional Nurse Coach Competencies

The Nurse Coach:

1. Involves the client in formulating goals that are specific, measurable, action-oriented, realistic, and time-lined.

2. Facilitates the client's process of self-discovery related to establishment of the client's goals.

3. Facilitates the client's exploration of alternative ideas and options relevant to goal-setting.

4. Supports the client's inner wisdom, intuition, and innate ability for knowing what is best for self.

5. Realizes that new goals will emerge as the client changes and evolves.

ANA Standard 4. Planning

The registered nurse develops a plan that prescribes strategies and alternatives to attain expected outcomes.

Professional Nurse Coach Role

The Nurse Coach and the client develop a coaching plan that identifies strategies to attain goals.

Professional Nurse Coach Competencies

The Nurse Coach:

1. Assists the client to identify strategies to attain goals.

2. Creates with the client an action plan with clearly defined steps and anticipated results.

3. Explores with the client potential obstacles to goal attainment and possible responses to these challenges.

4. Adjusts plan as desired by the client.

ANA Standard 5. Implementation

The registered nurse implements the identified plan.

Professional Nurse Coach Role

The Nurse Coach supports the client's coaching plan while simultaneously remaining open to emerging goals based on new insights, learning, and achievements. The Nurse Coach supports the client in reaching for new and expanded goals. The Nurse Coach utilizes a variety of specific coaching and communication skills to facilitate learning and growth.

Professional Nurse Coach Competencies

The Nurse Coach:

Before the coaching interaction:

1. Becomes fully present, centered, and grounded.

2. Reviews client status and/or progress from previously obtained data.

3. Minimizes distractions for self and encourages client to do the same.

At the beginning of the coaching interaction:

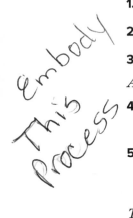

4. Explores, with the client, an outcome for the coaching session that is achievable in the time allotted.

5. Briefly explores progress since last coaching session, with particular attention to accomplishments, challenges, or barriers relevant to current session.

Throughout the coaching interaction:

6. Remains fully present, centered, and grounded.

   a. Supports the client in directing the agenda/focus of the coaching session.

   b. Acknowledges the client and identifies strengths for change.

   c. Maintains an interested, open, and reflective approach to the client.

   d. Is comfortable with silence or pausing to assist the client with reflection and finding new understanding or next steps.

   e. Accesses and trusts her/his own intuition and perceptions of the client.

   f. Draws upon the precepts of the human energy field/system to assist client in achievement of goals.

7. Creates a safe, supportive environment that fosters intimacy and trust.

8. Continuously exhibits authenticity (honesty, sincerity, personal integrity).

9. Demonstrates respect for client's subjective experiences/story, perceptions, learning style, and culture (e.g., beliefs, values, and customs).

10. Provides ongoing support for new ideas, behaviors, and actions that may involve risk-taking and fear of failure and/or fear of success. *whats scary about succeeding*

11. Obtains the client's consent to coach client in areas of vulnerability.

12. Chooses what is most effective in the moment from a variety of coaching strategies and implements as appropriate.

13. Focuses on what the client is saying and is not saying to understand the meaning in the context of the client's desires and to support the client's self-expression by employing such skills as deep listening, relevant use of language, powerful questioning, and direct communication.

    a. Deep Listening

       i. Accepts, explores, reinforces, and encourages the client's expression of perceptions, concerns, beliefs, suggestions, etc.

       ii. Recognizes incongruities between body language, words used, and the tone of voice.

       iii. Paraphrases, reiterates, and summarizes what the client has said to ensure understanding and clarity.

       iv. Focuses on the essence of the client's communication when the client becomes involved in long explanatory descriptions.

       v. Allows the client to express strong feelings without judgment in order to facilitate movement towards achievement of goals.

       vi. Acknowledges the client's ambivalence to change and helps identify barriers.

b. Relevant Use of Language

    i. Uses language, including metaphors and analogies, which assist the client to explore perspectives, uncertainties, or opportunities for change.

    ii. Uses language that is nonjudgmental, appropriate, and respectful.

    iii. Uses language that reflects the client's worldview, beliefs, and values.

c. Powerful Questioning

    i. Asks open-ended questions that create greater insight, clarity, and/or new possibilities and learning.

    ii. Asks questions that move the client towards desired goals.

    iii. Asks questions that evoke discovery, insight, commitment or action (e.g., those that challenge the client's assumptions).

    iv. Uses inquiry for greater awareness, clarity, and understanding.

d. Direct Communication

    i. Provides feedback in a clear and direct manner.

    ii. Shares insights with client in ways that are practical and meaningful.

    iii. Explores the client's assumptions and perspectives to evoke new ideas and discover new possibilities for action.

    iv. Challenges the client to stretch and be challenged, while maintaining a comfortable pace with the client.

14. Employs integrated, holistic communication skills including deep listening, relevant use of language, powerful questions, and direct communication, allowing the client to fully explore and articulate what she or he hopes to achieve through the coaching relationship.

    a. Supports the client's inner wisdom, intuition, and innate ability for learning.

    b. Identifies with the client additional areas for learning and development.

    c. Assists the client in uncovering underlying ambivalence, concerns, typical and fixed ways of perceiving self and the world, interpretations of experiences, and differences between thoughts, feelings, and actions.

    d. Helps the client identify barriers to change.

    e. Helps the client identify strengths and opportunities for learning and growth.

    f. Acknowledges client resistance as an opportunity for self-awareness and growth.

    g. Shares information with client that inspires broader perspectives.

    h. Encourages and supports the client to experiment and to apply what has been learned from the coaching interaction.

    i. Assists the client to determine actions that will enable the client to demonstrate, practice, and deepen new learning.

    j. Facilitates the client in taking action that will most effectively lead to achievement of desired goals and prevent relapse.

At the end of the coaching interaction:

15. Inquires of the client if the coaching session outcomes have been achieved.

16. Identifies the connection between where the client is and where she/he wishes to go.

17. Identifies with the client the next specific action steps and a timeline that will lead to achievement of desired goals.

18. Assists the client to manage progress by holding the client accountable for stated actions, results, and related time frames, while maintaining a positive and trusting relationship with the client.

19. Determines with the client when the next coaching interaction will occur.

20. Periodically, if relevant, prepares, organizes, and reviews information, including past and current actions, with the client that promotes achievement of client goals.

21. Periodically, as indicated, reviews and revises the coaching plan with the client.

22. Ends the coaching interaction in an energetic, positive, and supportive manner.

Reinforce their Role in success

ANA Standard 6. Evaluation

The registered nurse evaluates progress toward attainment of outcomes.

Professional Nurse Coach Role

The Nurse Coach partners with the client to evaluate progress toward attainment of goals.

Professional Nurse Coach Competencies

The Nurse Coach:

1. Assists the client to evaluate effectiveness of strategies in relation to the client's responses and the attainment of the expected and unfolding goals.

2. Supports client autonomy by recognizing the client is the determinant of progress and success.

3. Documents evaluation of progress and attainment of coaching goals.

Professional Nurse Coach Performance Competencies

ANA Standard 7. Ethics

The registered nurse practices ethically.

Professional Nurse Coach Role

The Nurse Coach integrates ethical provisions in all coaching interactions.

Professional Nurse Coach Competencies

The Nurse Coach:

1. Uses *Code of Ethics for Nurses with Interpretive Statements* (ANA, 2001) to guide practice and communicate the foundation of professional Nurse Coaching practice.

2. Clearly communicates to the client and others the distinctions among coaching, consulting, counseling, and teaching.

3. Provides coaching in a manner that recognizes and respects the client's autonomy, dignity, rights, values, and beliefs.

4. Maintains an effective coaching relationship that is congruent with the coaching agreement and within the boundaries of professional nursing practice.

5. Values all life experiences as opportunities to find personal meaning and cultivate self-awareness, self-reflection, and growth.

6. Maintains client confidentiality within legal and regulatory parameters.

ANA Standard 8. Education

The registered nurse attains knowledge and competence that reflects current nursing practice.

Professional Nurse Coach Role

The Nurse Coach attains knowledge and competence that reflects current Nurse Coaching practice.

Professional Nurse Coach Competencies

The Nurse Coach:

1. Participates in ongoing educational activities to enhance the Nurse Coaching role.

2. Documents and maintains evidence of Nurse Coaching competence.

3. Develops and uses a broad knowledge base related to holistic/integral nursing, integrative health, health systems, professional coaching competencies, counseling, health education, health promotion, and nursing practice issues.

ANA Standard 9. Evidence-Based Practice and Research

The registered nurse integrates evidence and research findings into practice.

Professional Nurse Coach Role

The Nurse Coach integrates evidence and research into Nurse Coaching practice.

Professional Nurse Coach Competencies

The Nurse Coach:

1. Uses the best available evidence, including theories and research findings, to guide and enhance professional Nurse Coaching practice.

2. Participates with others to establish research priorities and to identify research questions or areas for inquiry related to professional Nurse Coaching practice.

3. Participates in research activities related to professional Nurse Coaching practice.

ANA Standard 10. Quality of Practice

The registered nurse contributes to quality nursing practice.

Professional Nurse Coach Role

The Nurse Coach systematically enhances the quality and effectiveness of Nurse Coaching practice.

Professional Nurse Coach Competencies

The Nurse Coach:

Participates in quality improvement to enhance Nurse Coaching practice.

1. Contributes to the education of others concerning Nurse Coaching practice.

2. Documents Nurse Coaching interactions in a responsible, accountable, and ethical manner to facilitate quality review and promotion of effective Nurse Coaching practice.

3. Uses creativity and innovation in Nurse Coaching practice to improve client outcomes.

4. Analyzes organizational systems for barriers to effective implementation of Nurse Coaching practice.

5. Advocates use of *The Art and Science of Nurse Coaching: The Provider's Guide to Coaching Scope and Competencies* to evaluate and enhance the quality of practice.

ANA Standard 11. Communication

The registered nurse communicates effectively in a variety of formats in all areas of practice.

Professional Nurse Coach Role

The Nurse Coach employs skillful communication in all aspects of the coaching interaction.

Professional Nurse Coach Competencies

The Nurse Coach:

1. Understands that skillful communication is a fundamental component of professional Nurse Coaching practice.

2. Communicates, when requested by client, with family, significant others, caregivers, healthcare providers, and others to assist and enhance the client's achievement of coaching goals.

ANA Standard 12. Leadership

The registered nurse demonstrates leadership in the professional practice setting and the profession.

Professional Nurse Coach Role

The Nurse Coach demonstrates leadership in the promotion of effective Nurse Coaching for clients.

Professional Nurse Coach Competencies

The Nurse Coach:

1. Advances the role of the Nurse Coach among health professional and coaching colleagues and in professional organizations.

2. Develops cognitive, emotional, moral, and spiritual intelligence to enhance leadership skills.

3. Promotes the success of others by using effective Nurse Coaching interventions.

4. Demonstrates energy, excitement, and a passion for quality Nurse Coaching.

5. Willingly accepts that mistakes will be made by self and others when taking risks to achieve goals.

6. Displays the ability to define a clear vision, associated goals, and a plan to implement and measure progress toward goals.

ANA Standard 13. Collaboration

The registered nurse collaborates with healthcare consumer, family, and others in the conduct of nursing practice.

Professional Nurse Coach Role

The Nurse Coach collaborates with others to assist clients in achieving goals.

Professional Nurse Coach Competencies

The Nurse Coach:

1. Uses effective communication and change skills with individuals and groups to collaboratively identify and achieve individual, group, and organizational goals.

2. Works collaboratively with other health and wellness coaches in interprofessional development initiatives.

3. Collaborates with others to promote Nurse Coaching as a way to enhance client outcomes.

ANA Standard 14. Professional Practice Evaluation

The registered nurse evaluates her or his own nursing practice in relation to professional practice standards and guidelines, relevant statutes, and regulations.

Professional Nurse Coach Role

The Nurse Coach evaluates her or his own Nurse Coaching practice in relation to professional practice standards and guidelines, relevant statutes, rules, and regulations. The Nurse Coach is engaged in ongoing personal and professional self-development.

Professional Nurse Coach Competencies

The Nurse Coach:

1. Utilizes *The Art and Science of Nurse Coaching: The Provider's Guide to Coaching Scope and Competencies* to evaluate and enhance quality of practice.

2. Considers the effect of one's personal values, culture, spiritual beliefs, experiences, biases, and education on the provision of Nurse Coaching services to individuals, groups, and organizations.

3. Provides Nurse Coaching services in a manner that is appropriate and sensitive to culture and ethnicity.

4. Engages in self-evaluation of Nurse Coaching practice on a regular basis, identifying areas of strength as well as areas in which additional development would be beneficial.

5. Obtains evaluative feedback regarding one's own coaching from clients, peers, and professional colleagues and takes appropriate action based upon the feedback.

6. Pursues professional Nurse Coach certification as a way to demonstrate competence and to promote the Nurse Coaching role to employers, clients, and the public.

7. Recognizes that Nurse Coaching practice is enhanced by ongoing self-development to promote physical, mental, emotional, social, moral, and spiritual well-being.

8. Receives personal and professional coaching to enhance quality of Nurse Coaching practice.

9. Integrates knowledge from research on coaching into practice.

ANA Standard 15. Resource Utilization

The registered nurse utilizes appropriate resources to plan and provide nursing services that are safe, effective, and financially responsible.

Professional Nurse Coach Role

The Nurse Coach considers factors related to safety, effectiveness, cost, and impact on practice in the planning and delivery of Nurse Coaching services.

Professional Nurse Coach Competencies

The Nurse Coach:

1. Evaluates factors such as safety, effectiveness, availability, cost and benefits, efficiencies, and impact on Nurse Coaching practice when suggesting options for the client that would result in the same expected outcome.

2. Assists the client, as appropriate, in identifying and securing appropriate and available services to facilitate achievement of client goals.

ANA Standard 16. Environmental Health

The registered nurse practices in an environmentally safe and healthy manner.

Professional Nurse Coach Role

The Nurse Coach considers the impact of the internal and external environment of self and client when providing Nurse Coaching services.

Professional Nurse Coach Competencies

The Nurse Coach:

1. Understands that healthy environments encompass both internal and external environments

2. Recognizes that individual (physical, psychological, emotional, spiritual) and cultural, social, and historical factors influence internal and external environments.

3 Considers the internal and external healing environments of self and client regarding contribution to client goal achievement.

Glossary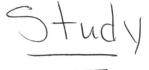

Source: Used with permission and adapted from Dossey & Keegan, 2013.

Active imagination. A process of conscious formation of images by the client as a technique or method to access deeper information and personal wisdom to facilitate changes; may include guided imagery.

Bearing witness. Being present for things as they are with the client or another; a state and skills that are achieved and learned through reflective practice (relaxation, prayer, meditation, nature walks) that can shift an experience of separateness to one of connection; it involves developing the qualities of stillness in order to be present for others.

Deep listening. The communication between two or more individuals in which the conventional division of self and ego is transcended by a sense of indivisible unity between all involved. Deep listening involves being present, allowing space and being focused with intention to understand what another person is expressing or not expressing (Dossey, Luck, & Schaub, 2013).

Emotional intelligence. The ability to perceive emotion in self and others; the ability to use emotions as a source of information; the ability to comprehend the complex relationships among emotions; and the ability to manage emotions to achieve desired outcomes. Emotional intelligence is concerned with understanding self and others and being able to relate to others. Emotional intelligence requires attunement to social norms. Emotional intelligence is a learned capability.

Environment. The context of habitat within which all living systems participate and interact, including the physical body and its physical habitat along with the cultural, psychological, social, and historical influences; includes both the external physical space and the person's internal physical, mental, emotional, social, and spiritual experience.

Environmental determinants of health. Any external agent (biological, chemical, physical, social, or cultural) that can be linked to a change in health status that is involuntary, i.e. breathing unwanted secondhand smoke, whereas active tobacco smoking is a behavioral determinant.

Ethics. The basic underlying concept of the unity and integral wholeness of all people and all of nature, identified and pursued by finding unity and wholeness within the self and within humanity. In this framework, acts are not performed for the sake of law, precedent, or social norms, but rather from a desire to do good freely in order to witness, identify, and contribute to unity.

Evidence-based practice. The process by which healthcare practitioners make clinical decisions using the best philosophy and theories, research evidence, clinical expertise, and patient preferences within the context of available resources.

Healing. The lifelong journey seeking harmony and balance in one's own life and in one's family, community, and global relations. Healing involves those physical, mental, social, and spiritual processes of recovery, repair, renewal, and transformation that increase wholeness and often (though not invariably) order and coherence. Healing is an emergent process of the whole system bringing together aspects of one's self and the body-mind-emotion-spirit-environment at deeper levels of inner knowing, leading toward integration and balance, with each aspect having equal importance and value. Healing can lead to more complex levels of personal understanding and meaning, and may be synchronous but not synonymous with curing. It is a sense of contentment with what is and a freedom from struggle.

Healing intention. The conscious awareness of being in the present moment to help facilitate the healing process; a volitional act of unconditional love.

Healing process. A continual journey of changing and evolving of one's self through life that is characterized by the awareness of patterns that support or are challenges/barriers to health and healing. This journey may be done alone or in a healing community. The healing process may occur until a person's final breath.

Healing relationships. The quality and characteristics of interactions between two people towards harmony and balance such as empathy, caring, love, warmth, trust, confidence, credibility, competence, honesty, courtesy, respect, sharing expectations, and a heart-to-heart connection.

Health. An individually defined state or process in which the individual (nurse, person, family, group, or community) experiences a sense of growth, well-being, harmony, and unity such that subjective experiences about health, health beliefs, and values are honored; a process of becoming an expanding consciousness.

Health promotion. Activities and preventive measures to facilitate growth, promote health, increase well-being, and actualize human potential of people, families, communities, society, and ecology such as immunizations, fitness/exercise programs, breast self-exams, appropriate nutrition, relaxation, stress management, social support, prayer, meditation, healing rituals, cultural practices, and promotion of environmental health and safety.

Holistic. Based on an understanding that patient is an interconnected unity and that physical, mental, emotional, social, spiritual, and environmental factors need to be included in any interventions. The whole is a system that is greater than the sum of its parts.

Holistic communication. A free flow of verbal and nonverbal interchange between and among people and significant beings such as pets, nature, and God/Life Force/Absolute/Transcendent that explores meaning and ideas leading to mutual understanding and growth.

Human caring. The moral ideal of nursing in which the nurse brings one's entire self into a relationship with the whole self of the client in order to protect the client's vulnerability, preserve her or his humanity and dignity, and reinforce the meaning and experience of oneness and unity.

Integral. A comprehensive synthesizing framework or multidimensional perspective. An integral approach addresses all levels of human experience (subjective and objective; individual and collective) in a combined, synergistic manner.

Integrative. An approach that puts the client at the center and addresses the whole person and full range of physical, emotional, mental, social, spiritual and environmental influences that affect health; includes the client's personalized action plan to maintain optimal health behaviors and human flourishing, and to heal illness and disease.

Intuition. The perceived knowing of things and events without the conscious use of rational processes; using all the senses to receive and process information.

Moral intelligence. The mental capacity to apply universal human principles, such as integrity, responsibility, compassion and forgiveness, to personal values, goals, and actions.

Not-knowing. Being free of fixed ideas.

X **Nurse Coach.** A registered nurse who integrates coaching competencies into any setting or specialty area of practice to facilitate a process of change or development that assists individuals or groups to realize their potential.

X **Nurse Coaching.** A skilled, purposeful, results-oriented, and structured relationship-centered interaction with clients provided by registered nurses for the purpose of promoting achievement of client goals.

X **Nurse Coaching process.** An iterative process that involves six steps that may occur simultaneously. (1) Establish relationship and assess client readiness for change; (2) Identify opportunities and issues; (3) Assist client to establish goals; (4) Structure the coaching interaction; (5) Empower clients to reach goals, and; (6) Assist client to determine extent to which goals were achieved.

Presence. The condition of being consciously and compassionately in the present moment with another, believing in her or his inherent wholeness, whatever the current situation; the essence of nursing care; the gift of self. Presence involves: approaching an individual or a situation in a way that respects and honors; relating in a way that reflects a quality of being with and in collaboration with; entering into a shared experience (or field of consciousness) that promotes growth, healing, and an experience of well-being. Presence is a combination of attributes that include intentionality, mutuality, client centeredness, and attending. Presence is a nursing intervention. Presence transforms experiences, adds a deeper, more powerful dimension, reduces anxiety and promotes a nurturing atmosphere. Presence is trying to understand the meaning of an experience for another without judgment. Presence is a way of being that involves connection so that growth and healing are promoted for self and others. Presence is necessary for genuine and empathetic communication.

Social determinants of health. The economic and social conditions under which individuals live that affect their health; disease and illness are often a result of detrimental social, economic, and political forces.

Spiritual intelligence. The recognition that physical reality is embedded within a larger, multidimensional reality with which we interact, knowingly or unknowingly. This larger reality includes and transcends the ego and the physical body. Spiritual intelligence involves the ability to act with compassion and wisdom, while maintaining inner and outer peace, regardless of circumstances. Spiritual intelligence includes the ability to access one's deepest meanings and highest motivations. It is the intelligence we use to determine that one course of action is more meaningful than another.

Suffering. An individual's experience of struggle based on a reinforced story around anxiety, distress, or pain. It can manifest as behavioral, emotional, mental, moral, physical, social and/or spiritual signs of distress; it is anguish experienced—internally and externally—as a threat to one's composure, integrity, sense of self, or the fulfillment of expectations.

Transpersonal. A personal understanding that is based on one's experiences of temporarily transcending or moving beyond one's usual identification with the limited biological, historical, cultural, and personal self at the deepest and most profound levels of experience possible. From this perspective the ordinary, biological, historical, cultural,. and personal self is seen as an important but only a partial manifestation or expression of this much greater something that is one's deeper origin and destination. It is that which transcends the limits and boundaries of individual ego identities and possibilities to include acknowledgment and appreciation of something greater (Schaub & Schaub, 2013).

Wellness. A desirable quality of life that provides satisfaction; a multidimensional state of existence experienced as well-being; integrated, congruent functioning aimed toward reaching one's highest potential.

Vulnerability. A universal human awareness that our physical lives are transitory; an awareness that can serve as a bridge among all peoples (Schaub & Schaub, 1997).

References

American Association of Colleges of Nursing (AACN). (2011). *Fact sheet.* Retrieved from: http://www.aacn.nche.edu/Media/FactSheets/nursfact. htm

American Holistic Nurses Association and American Nurses Association (AHNA/ANA). (2013). *Holistic nursing: Scope and standards of practice.* (2nd ed.) Silver Spring, MD: Nursesbooks.org.

American Holistic Nurses Credentialing Corporation (AHNCC). AHNCC Nurse Coach Certification. Retrieved from http://www.ahncc.org/ certification/nursecoachnchwnc.html

American Nurses Association (ANA) (2001.) *Code of Ethics for Nurses with interpretive statements.* Washington, DC: Nursesbooks.org.

American Nurses Association (ANA). (2010a). *Nursing: Scope and standards of nursing practice* (2nd ed.) Silver Spring, MD: Nursesbooks.org.

American Nurses Association (ANA). (2010b). *Nursing's social policy statement: The essence of the profession.* Silver Spring, MD: Nursesbooks. org.

Antonovsky, A. (1996). The salutogenic model as a theory to guide health promotion. *Health Promotion International, 11*(1), 11–18.

Atkinson, P. A., Martin, C. R., & Rankin, J. (2009). Resilience revisited. *Journal of Psychiatric and Mental Health Nursing, 16,* 137–145.

Baldwin, C. M., Schultz, A. A., Melnyk, B. M., & Rycroft-Malone, J. (2013). Evidence-based nursing practice. In B.M. Dossey & L. Keegan, *Holistic Nursing: A Handbook for Practice* (6th ed.), (pp. 797–814). Burlington, MA: Jones & Bartlett Learning.

Bandura, A. (1977). Self-efficacy: Toward a unifying theory of behavioral change. *Psychological Review* 84(2), 191, 215.

Bark Coaching Institute. (n.d.). *A path to learning successful coaching.* Retrieved from http://www.barkcoaching.com/coaching.html

Bark L. (2011). *The wisdom of the whole: Coaching for joy, health, and success.* San Francisco, CA: Create Space.

Barrett, E. A. M. (1983). *An empirical investigation of Martha E. Rogers' principle of helicy: The relationship of human field motion and power.* Unpublished doctoral dissertation, New York University, New York.

Barrett, E. A. M. (1989). A nursing theory of power for nursing practice: Derivation from Rogers' paradigm. In J. Riehl (Ed.). *Conceptual models for nursing practice* (3rd ed.). (pp. 207–217). Norwalk, CT: Appleton & Lange.

Barrett, E.A.M. (2003). Update on a measure of power as knowing participation in change. In O. L. Strickland & C. DiIorio (Eds.), Vol. 4. *Measurement of nursing outcomes: Focus on patient/client outcomes* (pp. 21–39). New York: Springer.

Becker, M. (1990). Theoretical models of adherence and strategies for improving adherence. In S. A. Shumaker, E.B. Schron, & J. K. Ockene (Eds.), *The handbook of human health behavior* (pp. 5–43). New York: Springer.

Benner, P. (1985). The oncology clinical specialist: An expert coach. *Oncology Nursing Forum 12*, 40–4.

Benner, P. (1984), *Novice to expert: Excellence and power in clinical nursing practice.* Menlo Park, CA: Addison-Wesley.

Carper, B. A, (1978). Fundamental patterns of knowing in nursing. *Advances in Nursing Science 1*(1), 13–23.

CGFNS International. Retrieved from http://www.cgfns.org/sections/about/

Chenoweth, L., Gallagher, R. Sheriff, J. N., Donoghue, J., & Stein-Parbury, J. (2008). Factors supporting self-management in Parkinson's disease: Implications for nursing practice. *International Journal of Older People Nursing, 3,* 187–193.

Cooperrider, D. L. & Whitney, D. (2005). *Appreciative inquiry: A positive revolution in change.* San Francisco, CA: Berrett-Koehler.

Cooperrider, D. L., Whitney, D., & Stavros, J. M. (2005). *Appreciative inquiry handbook.* Brunswick, OH: Crown Custom.

Cowling, R. (2001). Unitary appreciative inquiry. *Advanced Nursing Science, 23*(4), 32–48.

Csikszentmihalyi, M. (1990). *Flow: The psychology of optimal experience.* New York: Harper and Row.

Dart, M.A. (2011). *Motivational interviewing in nursing practice.* Sudbury, MA: Jones and Bartlett Learning.

Donner, G., & Wheeler, M. (2009). *Coaching in nursing: An introduction.* Indianapolis, IN: International Council of Nursing & Sigma Theta Tau. Retrieved from: http://www.nursingsociety.org/Education/ ProfessionalDevelopment/Documents/Coaching%20and%20 Mentoring%20Workbook_STTI.pdf

Dossey, B. M. (2013). Nursing: Integral, integrative, and holistic—local to global. In B.M. Dossey & L. Keegan, *Holistic Nursing: A Handbook for Practice* (6th ed.), (pp.1–57). Burlington, MA: Jones & Bartlett Learning.

Dossey, B. M. (2009). Integral and holistic nursing: Local to global. In B.M. Dossey & L. Keegan, *Holistic Nursing: A Handbook for Practice* (5th ed.), (pp. 3–46). Sudbury, MA: Jones and Bartlett Learning.

Dossey, B. M. (2010). *Florence Nightingale: Mystic, visionary, healer.* Commemorative Edition. Philadelphia: F. A. Davis.

Dossey, B. M., & Hess, D. (in press). *Professional Nurse Coach core curriculum.* (Unpublished manuscript). Available from author.

Dossey, B. M., & Keegan, L. (2013). *Holistic nursing: A handbook for practice* (6th ed.). Burlington, MA: Jones and Bartlett Learning.

Dossey, B. M., Luck, S., & Schaub, B. G. (2013). *Nurse coaching in health and wellness.* Huntington, NY: Florence Press.

Dossey, B. M., Selanders, L. C., Beck , D. M., & Attewell, A. (2005). *Florence Nightingale today: Healing, leadership, global action.* Silver Spring, MD: Nursebooks.org.

Erickson, H. L. (Ed.). (2010). *Exploring the interface between the philosophy and discipline of holistic nursing: Modeling and Role-Modeling at work.* Cedar Park, TX: Unicorns Unlimited.

Erickson, E., Tomlin, E., & Swain, M. A. (1983/2009). *Modeling and role-modeling: A theory and paradigm for nursing.* Englewood Cliffs, NJ: Prentice-Hall.

Fawcett, J. (1995). *Analysis and evaluation of conceptual models of nursing* (3rded.). Philadelphia: F. A. Davis.

Freshwater, D., Taylor, B. J., & Sherwood, G.C. (Eds.). (2008). *The international textbook of reflective practice in nursing.* Chichester, United Kingdom: Wiley-Blackwell.

Gillespie, B. M., Chaboyer, W., & Wallis, M. (2007). Development of a theoretically derived model of resilience through concept analysis. *Contemporary Nurse, 25*(1–2), 124–135.

Hatweg, D. L. & Fleck, L. M. Dorothea Orem's self-care deficit theory. In Parker, M. E. & Smith, M. C. *Nursing theories and nursing practice* (3rd ed.) (121–145). Philadelphia: F. A. Davis.

Hayes, E., & Kalmakis, K. A. (2007). From the sidelines: Coaching as a nurse practitioner strategy for improving health outcomes. *Journal of the American Academy of Nurse Practitioners, 19*(11), 555–562.

Hess, D., Bark, L., & Southard, M. E. (2010, September). White paper: Holistic Nurse Coaching. *Summit on standards & credentialing of professional coaches in healthcare & wellness.* Paper presented to National Credentialing Team for Professional Coaches in Healthcare, Boston, MA. Retrieved from http://www.ahncc.org/holisticnursecoaching.html

Hess, D. & Dossey, B. M. (In press). *Nurse coaching: A review of the literature.* (Submitted as a white paper to American Holistic Nurses Credentialing Corporation on December 16, 2011.) Available from authors.)

Hyman, M., Ornish, D., & Roizen, M. (2009). Life style medicine: Treating the causes of disease. *Alternative Therapies, 15*(6), 12–14.

Institute of Medicine. (2010). *The future of nursing: Leading change, advancing health.* Washington, DC: National Academies Press. Retrieved from http://www.iom.edu/Reports/2010/The-Future-of-Nursing-Leading-Change-Advancing-Health.aspx

Integrative Nurse Coach Certificate Program. (n.d.). *Why integrative nurse coaching?* Retrieved from http://inursecoach.com/education/why-inccp/

International Coaching Federation. (2011a), ICF core competencies. Retrieved from http://www.coachfederation.org/icfcredentials/core-competencies

International Coach Federation. (2011b). ICF stats. Retrieved from http://www.coachfederation.org/about-icf/press-room/

International Coaching Federation. (2011c). ICF Code of Ethics. Retrieved from http://www.coachfederation.org/icfcredentials/ethics/

International Council of Nurses. (n.d.)Retrieved from http://www.icn.ch/

Interprofessional Education Collaborative Expert Panel. (2011). *Core competencies for interprofessional collaborative practice: Report of an expert panel.* Washington, D.C.: Interprofessional Education Collaborative.

Johns, C. (2010). Reflection as a way-of-being in practice. In H. L. Erickson (Ed.), *Modeling and role-modeling at work,* (pp. 311–328). Cedar Park, TX: Unicorns Unlimited.

Kegan, R. & Lahey, L. L. (2009). *Immunity to change: How to overcome it and unlock the potential in yourself and your organization.* Boston: Harvard Business School Publishing.

Kimball, B., Joynt, J., Cherner, D., & O'Neil, E. (2007). The quest for new innovative care delivery models. *Journal of Nursing Administration 37*(9), 392–398.

Koerner, J. (2011). *Healing: The essence of nursing*. New York: Springer.

Kreitzer, M. J., Sierpina, V. S., & Lawson, K. (2008). Health coaching: Innovative education and clinical programs emerging. *Explore, 4*(2), 154–155.

Langeland, E., Wahl, A. K., Kristoffersen, K., & Hanestad, B. R. (2007). Promoting coping: Salutogenesis among people with mental health problems. *Issues in Mental Health Nursing, 28*, 275–295. doi: 10.1080/01612840601172627

Lawson, K. (2009). Could health coaching build a bridge to a new system of healthcare? *Alternative Therapies in Health and Medicine, 15*(5), 16–18.

Luck, S. (2010). Changing the health of our nation: The role of nurse coaches. *Alternative Therapies in Health and Medicine, 16*(5), 78–80.

McCraty R & Childres D. (2010). Coherence: Bridging personal, social, and global health. *Alternative Therapies in Health and Medicine*, 16(4), 10–24.

Mallock, K., & Porter-O'Grady, T. (2005). *The quantum leader: Applications for the new world of work*. Sudbury, MA: Jones and Bartlett.

McNally, K., & Cunningham, L. (2010). *Nurse executive's coaching manual*. Indianapolis, IN: Sigma Theta Tau International.

Meyers, D., Peikes, D., Genevro, J., Peterson, G., Taylor, E. F., Lake, T., & Grumbach, K. (2010). The roles of patient-centered medical homes and accountable care organizations in coordinating patient care. AHRQ Publication No. 11-M005-EF. Rockville, MD: Agency for Health Care Research and Quality. Retrieved from http://www.ahrq.gov/

Miller, W. R., Rollnick, S. (2002). *Motivational interviewing: Preparing people for change* (2nd ed.). New York: Guilford Press.

Moore, M. & Tschannen-Moran B. (2010). *Coaching psychology manual*. Philadelphia: Lippincott, Williams & Wilkins.

Moore, S. M., & Charvat, J. (2007). Promoting health behavior change using appreciative inquiry: Moving from deficit models to affirmation models of care. *Family and Community Health/Supplement 1, 30*(15), 564–574.

Munhall, P. L. (1993). Unknowing: Toward another pattern of knowing in nursing. *Nursing Outlook 41* (3), 125–128.

National Consortium for the Credentialing of Health and Wellness Coaches. (NCCHWC). 2010. National Summit on Standards and Credentialing of Professional Coaches in Healthcare and Wellness. September 26-27, 2010. Retrieved from http://www.ncchwc.org/files/SummitSundayPPT.pdf

National Consortium for the Credentialing of Health and Wellness Coaches (NCCHWC). (2011) *Progress report.* July. Retrieved from http://www. wellcoaches.com/images/pdf/progressreport-nationalteam-jul-2011.pdf

National Prevention Council (2011). *National Prevention Strategy: American's plan for better health and wellness.* Washington, DC: U.S. Department of Health and Human Services, Office of the Surgeon General. Retrieved from http://www.cdc.gov/policy/nps/

National Prevention Council (2012). *National Prevention Council Action Plan* Washington, DC: U.S. Department of Health and Human Services, Office of the Surgeon General. (2012). Retrieved from http://www.cdc. gov/policy/nps/

Newman, M. A. (1986). *Health as expanding consciousness.* St. Louis, MO: C.V. Mosby.

Newman, M. A. (1994). *Health as expanding consciousness.* (2nd ed.). St. Louis, MO: C.V. Mosby.

Neuman, B., & Fawcett, J. (Eds.). (2010). *The Neuman Systems Model* (5th ed.). Upper Saddle River, NJ: Pearson.

Nightingale, F. (1859). *Notes on hospitals.* London, England: John W. Parker.

Nightingale, F. (1860). *Notes on nursing: What it is and what it is not.* London, England: Harrison.

Nightingale, F. (1893). Sick-nursing and health-nursing. In B. Coutts (Ed.), *Woman's Mission* (pp. 184–205). London, England: Sampson, Low, Marston.

Nightingale Declaration for a Healthy World. Retrieved from http://www. nightingaledeclaration.net/the-declaration

Nursing Interventions Classification (NIC) (n.d.). NIC labels and definitions. Retrieved from http://www.nursing.uiowa.edu/cncce/nic-labels-and-definitions [Source: Bulechek, G.M., Butcher, H. K., & Dochterman, J.C. (Eds.). (2008). *Nursing Interventions Classification (NIC)* (5th ed.). St. Louis, MO: Mosby Elsevier.]

Orem, D. E. (1971). *Nursing concepts of practice*. New York: McGraw Hill.

Patient Protection and Affordable Care Act, H. R. 3590. Pub. L. No. 111–148 (2010). Retrieved from http://democrats.senate.gov/pdfs/reform/patient-protection-affordable-care-act-as-passed.pdf

Parse, R. R. (1981). *Man-living-health: A theory of nursing*. New York: John Wiley and Sons.

Parse, R. R. (1995). *Illuminations: The human becoming theory in practice and research*. New York: National League for Nursing Press.

Peplau, H. E. (1952). *Interpersonal relations in nursing*. New York: G. P. Putnam's Sons.

Potter, P., & Frisch, N. C, (2013). The nursing process. In Dossey, B. M. & Keegan, L. *Holistic nursing: A handbook for practice* (6th ed.) (145–160). Burlington, MA: Jones and Bartlett Learning

Prochaska, J.O., Norcross, J.C., & DeClemente, C.C. (1995). *Changing for good: A revolutionary six-stage program for overcoming bad habits and moving your life positively forward*. New York: Harper Collins.

Rogers, M. E. (1970). *An introduction to the theoretical basis of nursing*. Philadelphia, PA: F. A. Davis.

Rollnick, S., Miller, W.R., & Butler, C. C. (2008). *Motivational interviewing in healthcare: Helping patients change behavior*. New York: Guilford Press.

Roy, C. (2009). *The Roy Adaptation Model* (3rd ed.) Upper Saddle River, NJ: Prentice-Hall Health.

Samueli Institute. (2008). *Wellness initiative for the nation*. Alexandria, VA: Author. Retrieved from http://www.samueliinstitute.org/health-policy/wellness-initiative-for-the-nation-win

Schaub, B. G., Luck, S., & Dossey, B. M. (2012). Integrative nurse coaching for health and wellness. *Alternative and Complementary Therapies, 18*(1), 14–20.

Schaub, B.G. & Schaub, R. (1997). *Healing addictions: The vulnerability model of recovery.* Albany, NY: Delmar Publishers.

Schaub, R., & Schaub, B.G. (2009). *The end of fear: A spiritual path for realists.* Carlsbad, CA: Hay House.

Schaub, R. & Schaub, B. G. (2013). *Transpersonal development: Cultivating the human resources of peace, wisdom, purpose and oneness.* Huntington, NY: Florence Press.

Scholle, S.H., Torda, P., Peikes, D., Han, E., & Genevro, J. (2010). *Engaging patients and families in the medical home.* AHRQ Publication No. 10-0083-EF. Rockville, MD: Agency for Health Care Research and Quality. Retrieved from http://www.ahrq.gov/

Schenck, S. (2002). Nurse coach: Healthcare resource for this millennium. *Nursing Forum, 37*(3), 14–20.

Seligman, M. E. P. (1990). Learned optimism: How to change your mind and your life. New York: Free Press.

Sigma Theta Tau International. (n.d.)Retrieved from http://www. nursingsociety.org/aboutus/mission/Pages/factsheet.aspx

Southard, M. E. (2003). *A new provider for the new healthcare industry: The Nurse Coach.* (Unpublished manuscript). Available from author.

Snyderman, R., & Dinan, M. (2010). Improving health by taking it personally. *Journal of the American Medical Association, 303*(4), 363–364.

United Nations. (2011). Millennium Development Goals Report 2011. Retrieved from http://www.un.org/millenniumgoals/

U.S. Department of Health and Human Services, Office of Disease Prevention and Health Promotion, (n.d.). Introducing Healthy People 2020. Retrieved from http://www.healthypeople.gov/2020/about/default.aspx

Warelow, E. K. (2005). Resilience: When coping is emotionally intelligent. *Journal of the American Psychiatric Nurses Association, 11*(2), 101–2.

Watson Caring Science Institute. (n.d.). *Caritas coaching education program.* Retrieved from http://www.watsoncaringscience.org/index.cfm/category/3/caritas-coach-education-program-ccep.cfm

Watson, J. (1985). *Nursing: Human science and human caring: A theory of nursing.* Norwalk, CT: Appleton and Lange.

Watson, J. (2007). *Nursing human science and human care: A theory of nursing.* Sudbury, MA: Jones and Bartlett Learning.

White, J. (1995). Patterns of knowing: Review, critique, and update. *Advances in Nursing Science* 17(2), 73–86.

Wilson, M. (2009). Complexity theory. *Whitireia Nursing Journal,* (16), 18–24.

Wolever, R. Q., & Eisenberg, D. M. (2011). What is health coaching anyway? Standards needed to enable rigorous research. *Archives of Internal Medicine.* doi:10.1001/archinternmed.2011.508. Retrieved from http://archinte.jamanetwork.com/article.aspx?articleid=1106048

World Health Organization. (2009). *World Health Organization statistics report 2009.* Retrieved from http://www.learningnurse.com/content/view/34/49/

World Health Organization. (2011). United Nations high-level meeting on noncommunicable disease prevention and control, September 2011. Retrieved from www.who.int/nmh/publications/ncd_profiles2011/en/index.html

World Health Organization. (n.d.) Global Network of WHO Collaborating Centres (WHOCCs). Retrieved from http://www.parlatore.com.br/whocc/

Zahourek, R. P. (2013). Holistic nursing research: Challenges and opportunities. In B. M. Dossey & L. Keegan, *Holistic nursing: A handbook for practice* (6th ed.), (pp. 775–796). Burlington, MA: Jones & Bartlett Learning.

Appendix A.

Background

Formation of the Professional Nurse Coaching Workgroup (PNCW)

The Art and Science of Nurse Coaching: The Provider's Guide to Coaching Scope and Competencies is the product of significant exploratory conversations and electronic mail communication among the Professional Nurse Coach Workgroup (PNCW) (see the Contributors section for the members of this workgroup) over a three-year period and involving a six-step process.

Clarifying the Role of the Nurse Coach

During the initial PNCW meetings, foundational concepts of Nurse Coaching and the Nurse Coach role as a component of nursing practice were discussed. These discussions also included the growing emergence of nonprofessional health and wellness coaches as well as the development of health and wellness coaches in other professions. In September 2010, the PNCW circulated *White Paper on Holistic Nurse Coaching* (Hess, Bark, & Southard, 2010). All PNCW members attended the National Summit on Standards and Credentialing of Professional Coaches in Healthcare and Wellness (NCCHWC) convened by the National Consortium for the Credentialing of Health and Wellness Coaches Progress Report in Boston, Massachusetts, in Boston, Massachusetts, to explore the future of health and wellness coaches (NCCHWC, 2010; 2011). *The Art and Science of Nurse Coaching* has been developed by nurse coaching experts and vetted via a thorough peer-review process to fully describe the professional Nurse Coach role.

Initiating Nursing Alliances

The PNCW entered into a conversation regarding the importance of the role of the Nurse Coach and the need for a national certification process for Nurse Coaches with the American Holistic Nurse Credentialing Corporation (AHNCC). After lengthy discussion, the PNCW entered an agreement with

AHNCC whereby AHNCC would sponsor the work of the PNCW in exchange for the rights to establish a national certification process for the Nurse Coach. The Nurse Coach Certification process is voluntary. Nurses integrate Nurse Coach competencies in accordance with *Nursing: Scope and Standards of Practice*, 2nd Edition (ANA, 2010a). (See Appendix B.)

The PNCW and many nurse leaders continued to be engaged in conversations related to alliances with other interprofessional organizations (Interprofessional Education Collaborative Expert Panel, 2011; NCCHWEC, 2011) (see Steps 4 and 5 below) for the purpose of establishing clear guidelines and competencies for professional health and wellness coaches.

Articulating the Nurse Coach's Scope of Practice and Competencies and Six-Step Process

The creation of *The Art and Science of Nurse Coaching* is the successful completion of a three-year process. The PNCW engaged with a Review Committee and an Advisory Committee. (For the individuals who served on these and other groups involved in the process, see the Contributors section on pages vii and viii.) The following describes the extensive six-step course of action.

Step 1: Literature Review

The six-member PNCW conducted an extensive literature review regarding Nurse Coaching from 2009–2011. The goals were to: (1) Identify how the health and wellness coach role was embedded in nursing practice; (2) Identify areas where Nurse Coaching skills were used and integrated; (3) Determine how Nurse Coaches defined their roles, practices, and competencies; (4) Explore emerging trends within professional Nurse Coaching practice; and (5) Identify areas of future research in Nurse Coaching.

Step 2: The Compilation Process

Following Step 1 and during 2010–2011, the six-member PNCW compiled and reviewed the literature and discussed findings. Following a series of meetings, they drafted *Professional Nurse Coach Role: Defining Scope of Practice and Competencies*. The current retitled document is the result of extensive reviews and several revisions by the PNCW members.

Concurrently, and in preparation for Steps 3 and 4, the PNCW compiled a list of expert nurses engaged in coaching for the Review Committee and for the Advisory Committee.

Step 3: Review Committee

The expert Review Committee was provided with *The Art and Science of Nurse Coaching* and was directed to review and strengthen the document by providing additional comments, deletions, modifications, and recommendations. The revised draft document was again sent to the Review Committee for additional comments, deletions, modifications, and recommendations.

Step 4: Advisory Committee

The Advisory Committee was also provided with *The Art and Science of Nurse Coaching* and followed the same process as the Review Committee. The PNCW directive to the Advisory Committee also included the identification of strategies to obtain national and global nursing organizations endorsement (Step 5).

Step 5: Steps Toward Official ANA Document and Endorsing Organizations

The revised draft of *The Art and Science of Nurse Coaching* was sent to ANA on December 1, 2011 to begin the steps towards an officially recognized ANA document. As soon as this process was completed (in early 2012) the document was sent to their 28 affiliate organizations. The PNCW has followed the recommendations of ANA and the Advisory Board regarding contact with other national and global nursing organizations. The CGFNS International was the first global endorsing organization. As organizations responded with endorsement they were added to the list that appears in the Contributors section on page ix.

Step 6: Development of Core Curriculum for Professional Nurse Coaching Practice

Following completion of each of the steps previously described, and in partnership with Nurse Coaching experts and endorsing organizations, *Professional Nurse Coach Core Curriculum* will be developed and published.

Background Summary

The Art and Science of Nurse Coaching brings one dimension of nursing's leadership role in healthcare reform to the forefront. This document will also assist nurses involved in interprofessional conversations related to the establishment of standards of practice and a credentialing process for health and wellness coaches (Kreitzer, Sierpina, & Lawson, 2008; Lawson, 2009; Moore & Tschannen-Moran, 2010; NCCHWC, 2011).

This document clarifies nursing perspectives concerning the role of the Nurse Coach in five key ways: (1) It specifies the philosophy, beliefs, and values of the Nurse Coach and the Nurse Coach's scope of practice; (2) It articulates the relationship between *The Art and Science of Nurse Coaching* and *Nursing: Scope and Standards of Practice*, 2nd Edition (ANA, 2010a); (3) It provides the basis for continued interdisciplinary conversations related to professional health and wellness coaches and lay health and wellness coaches; (4) It lays the foundation for an international certification process for professional Nurse Coaching practice; and (5) It identifies the need to develop a core curriculum for professional Nurse Coaching practice that can be used in practice, education, research, and healthcare policy.

Appendix B.

The American Holistic Nurses Credentialing Corporation (AHNCC) Nurse Coach Certification Process

Initiating Nursing Alliances

The PNCW entered into a conversation with the American Holistic Nurse Credentialing Corporation (AHNCC) regarding the paradigm shift toward health and wellness inherent in the Patient Protection and Affordable Care Act, and the importance of developing a role and certification program for the professional Nurse Coach. Given that holistic nurses specialize in the practice of health and wellness, it was mutually determined that AHNCC was the appropriate venue for a national certification program for professional Nurse Coaches. After lengthy discussion, the PNCW entered an agreement with AHNCC whereby AHNCC would sponsor the work of the PNCW in exchange for the rights to establish a national certification process for the Nurse Coach.

Certification Examination Development

AHNCC and the Professional Testing Corporation of New York (PTC) collaborated to develop a set of competencies extrapolated from the literature and in accordance with *Nursing: Scope and Standards of Practice*, 2nd ed. (ANA, 2010a). The competencies, reviewed by three expert panels, were revised until approved, and then used for a role-delineation study. The results from that role-delineation study were used to develop a Blueprint, and guide the development of the Nurse Coach certification examination.

A multiple-step process, overseen by PTC, was used to develop the examination including: item-writing to assess specified competencies, item-reviews to assess content validity, and an exam-development process to assess content and construct validity. An item-analysis step, to assess for reliability, is undertaken following the administration of each examination. The Nurse Coach examination will be piloted February, 2013. Additional information is available on the AHNCC website: www.ahncc.org or http://www.ahncc.org/certification/nursecoachnchwnc.html.

Appendix C.

The Nurse Coach Role in Healthcare Transformation

Appendix C documents the forces that catalyzed the initial grassroots work of six nurses to create this document and describes how the professional Nurse Coach role can contribute to national and global healthcare transformation.

Nurse Coaches in National Healthcare Transformation

Nurse Coaches can be leaders in engaging clients in self-care and adoption of healthy life style behaviors that lead to improved healthcare outcomes. A focus on transformation of health care is leading to new models of care delivery that incorporate the professional Nurse Coach role. In 23 of the 24 models discussed in *Innovative Care Delivery Models: Identifying New Models that Effectively Leverage Nurses* (Kimball, Joynt, Cherner, & ONeill, 2007), organizations created new roles for nurses that gave increased accountability for achieving successful patient quality, safety, and satisfaction outcomes. The concept of Nurse Coaches was also described as helping patients make successful transitions across settings.

In 2008, the Samueli Institute released its visionary report entitled *Wellness Initiative for the Nation (WIN)* (2008). This report advocated new approaches to health prevention and health promotion. Referring to a "broken disease treatment system" (p. 4), the authors stated that a new vision of health based upon human flourishing is needed. The report presented the idea of health coaches as one way to significantly reduce healthcare costs and mortality. They and others realized that current healthcare delivery practices, whether conventional or holistic, are in need of models of care that provide a wide range of choices for individuals that are efficient, effective, and reduce costs. This is fundamental to transforming health care from a disease-based model of care to one that focuses on health and wellness.

In March 2010, the Patient Protection and Affordable Care Act (PPACA) became law (HR3590) (Patient Protection and Affordable Care Act, 2010). The language in the PPACA refers to partnerships with a diverse group of licensed health professionals including practitioners of integrative health, preventive medicine, health coaching, public education, and more.

Many provisions in health care home and accountable care models are based on interprofessional care coordination that is patient-centered. The Agency for Healthcare Research and Quality (AHRQ) has funded and published projects that clearly address the need for a revitalized care system where decisions are based within the context of patient's values and preferences (Meyers et al., 2010). Asking patients and families what matters most to them is a critical step in engaging them in care. Coordinated patient-centered care that includes actively engaged patients requires a new set of skills for providers, patients, and families (Scholle, Torda, Peikes, Han, & Genevro, 2010).

In December 2010, the Healthy People 2020 initiative (U.S. Department of Health and Human Services, n.d.) was announced. This exhaustive, multiyear, collaborative process among the U.S. Department of Health and Human Services (HHS) and other federal agencies, public stakeholders, and the advisory committee continues the work started in 2000 with the Healthy People 2010 plan for improving the nation's health. (See also the discussion of Healthy People 2020 on pages 23 and 29.)

In June 2011, the National Prevention, Health Promotion, and Public Health Council announced the release of the National Prevention and Health Promotion Strategy, a comprehensive plan that will help increase the number of Americans who are healthy at every stage of life (National Prevention Strategy, 2011). The National Prevention and Health Promotion Strategy document addresses the importance of healthy foods, clean air and water, and safe worksites that is directly related to national and global healthcare transformation. (See also the discussion of the National Prevention Strategy in this document.)

Professional Nurse Coaches and Global Healthcare Transformation

To achieve global healthcare transformation, the United Nations Millennium Development Goals (MDGs), declared in 2000, must be achieved for the 21st century to progress toward a sustainable quality of life for all of humanity (United Nations, 2011). These eight MDGs are as follows:

- MDG 1. Eradicate Extreme Poverty and Hunger

- MDG 2. Achieve Universal Primary Education

- MDG 3. Promote Gender Equality and Empower Women

- MDG 4. Reduce Child Mortality

- MDG 5. Improve Maternal Health

- MDG 6. Combat HIV/AIDS

- MDG 7. Ensure Environmental Sustainability

- MDG 8. Develop Global Partnerships

These Goals are an ambitious agenda for improving lives worldwide. Of these eight, MDGs 4, 5, and 6 are directly related to health and nursing. The other five (MDGs 1, 2, 3, 7, and 8) are factors that determine the health or lack of health of people. For each goal, one target to be achieved by 2015 has been established, using 1990 data as a benchmark.

"Health" is the common thread that runs through all eight UN MDGs. Professional Nurse Coaches are part of the 17.6 million nurses and midwives of the world (WHO, 2009). They understand that these goals point directly back to the work Florence Nightingale achieved in her time (Nightingale Declaration for a Healthy World, n.d.). These goals are directly related to the work of all nurses everywhere, many of whom who are engaged in coaching people to find local solutions at the global level.

The leadership of professional Nurse Coaches can initiate new approaches to improved global health by empowering individuals and groups to carry Nightingale's legacy forward into the 21st century to address the environmental and social determinates of health. New efforts must be implemented to prevent disease and to create strategies for a healthy and fit world, recognizing that prevention must become part of daily life. This is the work of the four international organizations discussed next.

International Council of Nurses

The International Council of Nurses (ICN) is a federation of more than 130 national nurses associations that represent the millions of nurses worldwide (ICN, n.d.). Founded in 1899, ICN is the world's first and widest reaching international organization for health professionals. Operated by nurses, ICN works to ensure the quality of nursing care for all, sound health policies globally, the advancement of nursing knowledge, and the presence worldwide of a respected nursing profession and a competent and satisfied nursing workforce. Professional Nurse Coaches can contribute to the quality of nursing care, influence healthcare policy, and be involved in scientific advances.

Global Network of WHO Collaborating Centres for Nursing and Midwifery Development

To organize nursing and midwifery leadership, the Global Network of WHO Collaborating Centres (WHOCCs) for Nursing and Midwifery Development is an independent, international, non-for-profit, voluntary organization, currently comprising 44 institutions of excellence, from the six regions of the World Health Organization (WHO) (WHOCC, n.d.). Founded in 1988, the Network strives to enhance the collaborative activities of Nursing and Midwifery Collaborating Centres, supporting WHO's efforts towards Health for All (World Health Organization, 2011). Professional Nurse Coaches can include coaching skills in the provision of direct care. They can also advocate for the UN's MDG4 (Reduce Child Mortality), which is related to the health of infants. MDG 5 (Improve Maternal Health) sits at the core of one of today's most critical global health concerns. Clearly nursing practice has been and must continue to be integrally involved in this challenge.

CGFNS International

CGFNS International (also known as the Commission on Graduates of Foreign Nursing Schools) is to serve the global community through programs and services that verify and promote the knowledge-based practice competency of healthcare professionals. The Commission on Graduates for Foreign Nursing Schools (CGFNS) began in 1977. CGFNS has reviewed and/or certified the credentials of over 500,000 foreign-educated nurses and other healthcare professionals for U.S. licensure and immigration. The vision of CGFNS is to be the premier source of credentials evaluation and professional development services that provide strategic value and direction to healthcare professionals worldwide (CGFNS, n.d.). The Nurse Coach recognizes the importance of sound credentialing and deepening the professional development of the nurse.

Sigma Theta Tau International

The Honor Society of Nursing, Sigma Theta Tau International (STTI), founded in 1922 with 125,000 active members, has as its mission to support the learning, knowledge and professional development of nurses committed to making a difference in health worldwide (STTI, n.d.). The STTI vision is to create a global community of nurses who lead in using knowledge, scholarship, service and learning to improve the health of the world's people. The importance of the professional Nurse Coach role has been recognized by STTI, as evidenced by the organization's publication of *Coaching in Nursing* (Donner & Wheeler, 2009).

Appendix D.

Theories in Nurse Coaching Practice

Overview: Nursing Theories and Other Theories

Appendix D provides an overview of the recognized meta-paradigm in nursing and patterns of knowing with application to professional Nurse Coaching. It also discusses many frequently used nursing theories and other social theories in professional Nurse Coaching practice. The nursing theories discussed are Rogers' Theory of Science of Unitary Human Beings, Orem's Self-Care Deficit Nursing Theory, Roy's Adaptation Model, Neuman's Systems Model, Parse's Theory of Human Becoming, Barrett's Knowing Participation in Change Theory, Erickson's Theory of Modeling and Role-Modeling, Watson's Theory of Human Science and Human Care, Newman's Health as Expanding Consciousness Theory, and Dossey's Theory of Integral Nursing. Social science and other theories and concepts that are often used in Nurse Coaching include change theories, positive psychology, resilience, coherence theory, complexity science, energy theories, story theory, and reflective practice.

Nursing Meta-Paradigm and Patterns of Knowing and Its Application to Professional Nurse Coaches

Paradigms and worldviews can impact Nurse Coaches as they reflect on the nature of human beings, health, environment, and caring. Fawcett (1995) articulated four components recognized as the meta-paradigm in a nurse theory—nurse, person, health, and environment (society). Meta-paradigm definitions may vary in different nursing theories; however, the four domains are seen as interrelated and interdependent and each informs and influences the others.

As a way to organize nursing knowledge, Carper (Carper, 1978) in her now classic 1978 article, identified the four fundamental patterns of knowing (personal, empirics, ethics, aesthetics) followed by Munhall's (1993) introduction of the pattern of not knowing, and White's (1995) introduction of the pattern of sociopolitical knowing. These patterns continue to be refined and reframed with new applications and interpretations. Understanding these patterns of knowing can assist Nurse Coaches to bring themselves into the full expression of being present in the moment with self and others, to integrate aesthetics with science, and to develop the flow of ethical experience with thinking and acting.

Nursing Theories

Theory of Science of Unitary Human Beings

Martha Rogers (1970, 1994) was one of the first contemporary nurse scholars to articulate the idea that humans are whole beings and cannot be understood by reducing them to parts. "The descriptive, explanatory, and predictive principles that direct professional nursing practice are rooted in a fundamental concept of the wholeness of life" (Rogers, 1970, p. 34.) Her ideas, developed over several years, led to the development of the Science of Unitary Human Beings. Rogers' ideas encompassed a pan-dimensional and transcendent view of humans as ever evolving energy fields. Rogers encouraged nurses not to become stuck in present reality, but to look forward to envision how life might be in a universe where there is continuous change (Rogers, 1994).

Self-Care Deficit Nursing Theory   *Agency, Demand, Requsists*

Dorothea Orem's Self-Care Deficit Nursing Theory (SCDNT) was first published in 1971 and subsequently expanded through 2001 (Orem, 1971, Hartweg & Fleck, 2009). She saw people as individuals that should be self-reliant and responsible for their own care. Self-care and dependent care are behaviors that are learned within a socio-political context. A person's knowledge related to health and potential health problems is necessary to promote self-care behaviors. Nursing is a form of action and interaction between two or more individuals. Successfully meeting universal and development self-care requisites is an important component of primary care prevention. She defined self-care as the practice of activities that individuals initiate and perform to maintain life, health and well-being. Self-care agency implies a person's ability for engaging in self-care conditioned by age developmental state, life experiences, sociocultural orientation and available resources. Therapeutic self-care demand is described as the totality of self-care actions to be performed for some duration to meet the person's self-care requisites. Self-care requisites are any actions directed towards provision of self-care. Nursing is required when an individual (dependent) is unable or limited in the ability to provide continuous and effective care.

Adaption Model *Adaptation, Individual, Group, System*

Sister Callista Roy's (2009) model appeared in 1970 with an expansion in the mid-70s to the mid-80s. The Adaption Model major concepts include people as adaptive systems (both individuals and groups), environment, health, and the goal of nursing using the six-step nursing process. She views the individual as a set of interrelated, biological, psychological, and social systems. She believes that all individuals strive to maintain balance and cope with life's challenges, with each person having a unique style. It is this individual range of adaptability that determines how one deals with new experiences and challenges. There are four main adaptation systems: (1) the physiological-physical system, (2) the self-concept group identity system, (3) the role mastery/function system, and (4) the interdependency system. Roy's goal of nursing is the promotion of adaptation in each of the four modes that contribute to the individual's health, quality of life, and dignity in dying. Roy sees the person as a bio-psychosocial being constantly interacting with a changing environment. The person is an open system who uses coping skills to deal with life's problems and challenges. Health is the process of being and becoming an integrated and whole person. The environment is seen as all conditions and behaviors of the person. It is a universal model adaptable to numerous situations. The nurse's role is to promote system stability by using three levels of prevention.

Neuman Systems Model *Stress*

Betty Neuman (Newman & Fawcett, 2010) developed the Neuman Systems Model (NSM) in 1970 and was first published in 1974. She replaced the word *patient* with the word *client*. She views the client as a holistic being which physiological, psychological, sociological, and developmental aspects. This model is based on the client's relationship to stress, reaction to it, and reconstitution factors that are dynamic and changing.

Theory of Human Becoming *Unitary Whole, Presence*

Rosemarie Rizzo Parse (1981, 1995) developed the idea of the person as a unitary whole suggesting that the person can only be viewed as a unity. She describes nursing as a scientific discipline and the practice of nursing as an art in which nurses serve as guides to assist others in making choices affecting health. Person is a unified, whole being. Health is a process of becoming; it is a personal commitment, an unfolding, a process related to lived experiences. Environment is the universe. The human-universe is inseparable and evolving as one. The concept of "presence" is emphasized in this theory as a critically important nurse intervention.

Knowing Participation in Change Theory *Power Profile*

Elisabeth Barrett (1983, 1989, 2003) developed the Knowing Participation in Change Theory. Her power theory elaborates on Martha Rogers' (1970) axiom that humans can participate knowingly in change. She proposed that power is the capacity to participate knowingly in the nature of change characterizing the continuous mutual process of people and their world. Power as knowing participation in change is being aware of what one is choosing to do, feeling free to do it, and doing it intentionally. According to this theory, power is inherently value free. The observable, measurable dimensions of power are awareness, choices, freedom to act intentionally, and involvement in creating change. The inseparable association of the four power dimensions is termed a person's or group's Power Profile. The Power Profile is not static; it varies based on the changing nature of the human-environment mutual process of various individuals and/or groups. These changes indicate: (1) the nature of the awareness of experiences; (2) the type of choices made; (3) the degree to which freedom to act intentionally is operating; and (4) the manner of involvement in creating specific changes.

Modeling and Role-Modeling Theory

Helen Erickson and her colleagues (Erickson, Tomlin, & Swain, 1983/2009) published a theory and paradigm for nursing called the Modeling and Role-Modeling Theory that draws on work from many theoretical perspectives. In this theory there are five aims of all nursing interventions: (1) to build trust; (2) to promote positive orientation; (3) to promote perceived control; (4) to

Whole is Greater than Sum of Parts

promote strengths; and (5) to set mutual goals that are health-directed. The nurse uses this theory by creating a model of the client's world (*Modeling*) and then uses that model to plan interventions and to demonstrate and support health-producing behaviors from within the client's worldview (*Role Modeling*). This theory depicts nursing as a process that demands an interpersonal and interactive relationship with the client. Facilitation, nurturance, and unconditional acceptance must characterize the nurse's care giving. The human person is seen as a holistic being with interacting subsystems (biologic, psychological, social, and cognitive), and with an inherent genetic base and spiritual drive; the whole is greater than the sum of its parts (Erickson, 2010).

Theory of Human Science and Human Care *Transpersonal Caring*

Jean Watson (1985, 2007) emphasizes the relationship between two beings as fundamental for nursing practice: it must never be diminished or lost. Nursing's role in society is based on human caring. Caring is our moral imperative. Caring and loving are primal energetic forces; we all need to be loved and cared for. Transpersonal caring is a means of moving toward a higher sense of self and harmony with mind, body, and soul. Access to a higher sense of self is accessed through one's emotions and thoughts—the subjective inner world. Transpersonal caring allows humanity to grow towards greater harmony, spiritual evolution, and perfection. The transpersonal caring relationship depends upon: (1) a moral commitment to human dignity; (2) the nurse's intent and will to affirm the subjective significance of other; (3) the nurse's ability to detect feelings; (4) the nurse's ability to feel a union with another; and (5) the nurse's own history.

Health as Expanding Consciousness Theory *The Person is Consciousness*

Margaret Newman (1986, 1994) describes health as the expansion of consciousness. The theory of Health as Expanded Consciousness is grounded in Newman's personal experience and was stimulated by Rogers' (1970) description of the unitary nature of a human being in interaction with the environment. Health and illness is a single process moving through varying degrees of organization and disorganization, but all one unitary process. The total pattern of person-environment is a network of consciousness. Consciousness is everywhere. A person, rather than possessing consciousness, *is* consciousness. Consciousness is ever evolving, and "the process of evolution of consciousness is also the process of health" (Newman, 1986, p. 43). In Newman's model of health, there is no basis for rejecting any experience as irrelevant. The important factor is to become attuned to one's pattern of interaction and to recognize that it is one of expanding consciousness. The nurse practicing from this understanding "enters into a partnership with the client with the mutual goal of participating in an authentic relationship, trusting that in the process of evolving, both will grow and become healthier in the sense of higher levels of consciousness" (p. 68).

Theory of Integral Nursing   4 Quadrants

Barbara Dossey (2009, 2013) has developed her Theory of Integral Nursing, which includes an integral worldview and four perspectives of human experience and reality: (1) the individual interior; (2) the individual exterior; (3) the collective interior; and (4) the collective exterior. Each perspective is considered equally important. The Theory of Integral Nursing builds upon a solid holistic, integrated, and multidimensional theoretical nursing foundation and may be used with other integral and holistic nursing concepts, theories, and research. The integral approach allows nurses to more fully consider and comprehend the complexity of human experience. Healing is a core concept of the Theory of Integral Nursing. Healing is "the innate natural phenomenon that comes from within a person and describes the indivisible wholeness and the interconnectedness of all people, and all things" (Dossey, 2013, p. 27).

Change Theories

Behavioral change theories most frequently used in professional Nurse Coaching include the Transtheoretical Stages of Change Model (Prochaska, Norcross, & DeClemente, 1995), the Health Belief Model (Becker, 1990), Self-Efficacy (Bandura, 1977), Immunity to Change (Kegan & Lahey, 2009), and Motivational Interviewing (Dart, 2011; Miller & Rollnick, 2002; Rollnick, Miller, & Butler, 2008) and have been adopted by many Nurse Coaches (Hess et al., 2010). Concepts and strategies embedded within these approaches are applied in coaching interactions to promote self-efficacy and to uncover resistance and identify barriers to change. Appreciative Inquiry (Cooperrider & Whitney, 2005; Cooperrider, Whitney, & Stavros, 2005; Moore & Charvat, 2007) is another model of change that focuses on client strengths to create a more positive future, while Unitary Appreciative Inquiry (Cowling, 2001) is a related approach utilized by nurses to know the wholeness and uniqueness of each person as the context for change.

Positive Psychology

Positive psychology is a recent branch of psychology that places emphasis on ways to make normal life more fulfilling and focuses on strengths and human flourishing (Seligman, 1990; Csikszentmihalyi, 1990). Researchers study states of flow, values, strengths, virtues and talents and how these areas can be enhanced in social systems, organizations, and institutions. This field does not replace traditional psychology. At the *subjective level* the focus is on the positive subjective experience, which includes: well-being and satisfaction (past), and flow, joy, the sensual pleasures, and happiness (present), and constructive cognitions about the future-optimism, hope, and faith. At the *individual level* it is about positive individual traits: the capacity for love and vocation, courage, interpersonal skill, aesthetic sensibility, perseverance, forgiveness, originality, future-mindedness, high talent, and wisdom. At the *group level* it is about the civic virtues and the institutions that move individuals toward better citizenship: responsibility, nurturance, altruism, civility, moderation, tolerance, and work ethic.

Resilience

Resilience is generally considered to be a positive trait involving the capacity to cope with stress and adversity (McCraty & Childers, 2010). Resilience can be an outcome of good coaching and emerges from learned optimism (Seligman, 1990). *Physical resilience* is reflected in physical flexibility, endurance, and strength. *Mental resilience* is reflected in one's attention span, mental flexibility, optimistic worldview, and ability to integrate multiple points of view. *Emotional resilience* is related to one's ability to self-regulate the expression of one's emotions. *Spiritual resilience* is related to one's commitment to one's core values, the ability to trust one's intuition, and tolerance of others' values and beliefs. While questions remain concerning the development of resilience (Atkinson, Martin, & Rankin, 2009), there are nurse scholars who contend that development of resilience is a process that can be supported and developed at any time, and that development of resilience has the potential to improve clinical outcomes (Gillespie, Chaboyer, & Wallis, 2007; Warelow, 2005).

Sense-of-Coherence Theory

Salotogenesis

The Sense-of-Coherence (SOC) theory is a theory of salutogenesis. Developed by Antonovsky (1996), this theory represents a perspective that is different from a traditional pathogenic orientation of health. The focus is on what makes a person move towards health. "The focus is on the story of the person rather than the diagnosis. The person is understood as an open system in active interaction with the environment (both external and internal conditions)" (Langeland, Wahl, Kristoffersen, & Hanestad, 2007, p. 277). A sense of coherence concerns the extent to which one has a feeling of confidence that one's internal and external environments are predictable and can be explained. The Sense-of-Coherence theory contains three components: comprehensibility, manageability, and meaningfulness. Comprehensibility refers to the ability to understand situations. Manageability refers to a person's perception that needed resources are available. Meaningfulness refers to the extent to which life is perceived as making sense emotionally and is often considered the most important component (Langeland, et al, 2007). A sense of coherence will influence the motivation to engage in self-management of one's health (Chenworth, Gallagher, Sheriff, Donoghue, & Stein-Parbury, 2008).

Complexity Science   *All is connected, Change small increment*
Quantum or complexity science is a set of theoretical constructs that look at the universe as comprised of complex adaptive systems – as a set of interrelationships (Malloch & Porter-O'Grady, 2005). All is connected. Relationships between and among individuals and their collective relationships to systems create a complex whole. Change is achieved through small and successful increments that when aggregated lead to greater and broader change. The nonlinearity of complex adaptive systems favors continuous innovation and creativity over stability, strict formats, and unchanging structures. Nurses who can adapt and co-evolve with new situations as they emerge—who are able to focus on process, avoiding rigid goals and prescriptive content (Wilson, 2009)— are maximally positioned to be change facilitators. In quantum change, all process is dynamic and continuous; it neither begins nor ends. One moves in dance as conditions adapt and change, and change again. Underneath surface appearances lie chaos, unpredictability, paradox, and complexity—foundations upon which new order and symmetry will appear.

Reflective Practice   *Mindfulness*
Reflective practice is the process of developing new insights through self-awareness and critical reflection upon experiences – both past experiences and in-the-moment experiences (Freshwater, Taylor, & Sherwood, 2008). Reflective nursing practice involves the capacity to be open to different viewpoints and to recognize opportunities for change. "Being mindful is the quintessential nature of reflective practice" (Johns, 2010, p. 313). Being mindful involves being a witness without judgment; it transcends the rational mind and integrates all knowing.

Appendix E.

Interventions Frequently Used in Nurse Coaching Practice

Many of these interventions are listed in the current Nursing Interventions Classification system (NIC, n.d.).

- Affirmation
- Appreciative Inquiry
- Aromatherapy
- Art Therapy
- Celebration
- Client Assessments
- Cognitive Reframing
- Contracts
- Deep Listening
- Exercise
- Goal Setting
- Guided Imagery
- Holistic Self-Assessments
- Humor and Laughter
- Intention
- Journaling
- Meditation
- Mindfulness Practice

- Motivational Interviewing
- Movement
- Music and Sound Therapy
- Observation
- Play
- Powerful Questions
- Prayer
- Presence
- Probing Questions
- Reflection
- Relaxation Modalities
- Ritual
- Self-Care Interventions
- Self-Reflection
- Silence
- Somatic Awareness
- Stories
- Visioning

Index